Our Technology Issue

HOPE

October 2017

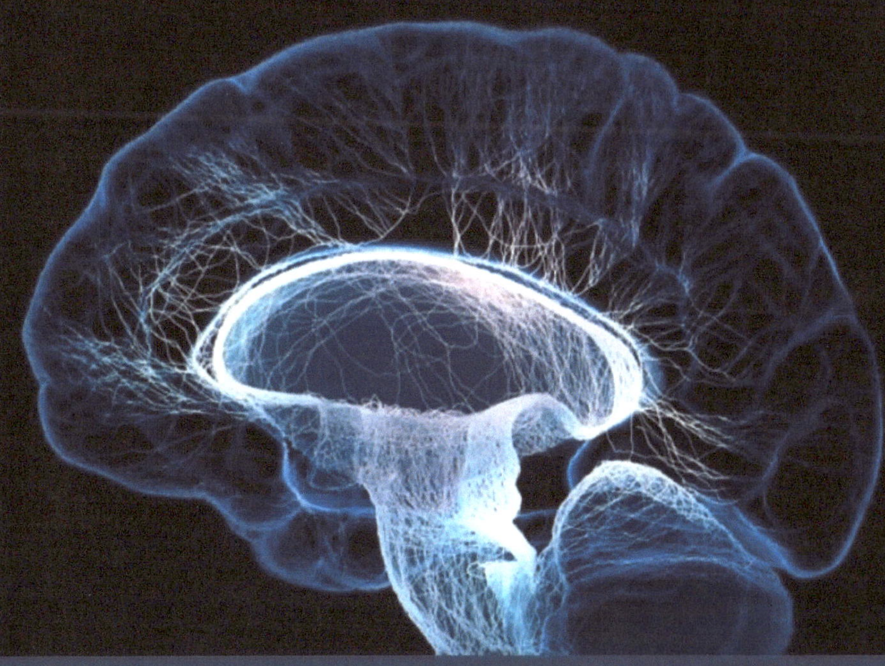

TBI
Advocacy & Education
HOPE
MAGAZINE

*"Supporting the
Brain Injury Community"*

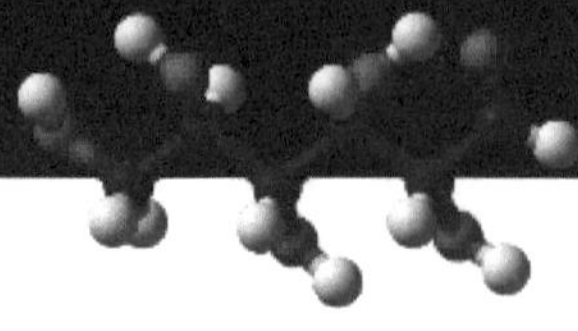

TBI HOPE MAGAZINE

Serving All Impacted by Brain Injury

October 2017

Publisher
David A. Grant

Editor
Sarah Grant

Contributing Writers
Pamela Donahoe
David A. Grant
Tristan Greenman
Derek O'Brien
Saba Rizvi
Jennifer Stokley
Arlene Weintraub

Amazing Cartoonist
Patrick Brigham

FREE subscriptions at
www.TBIHopeMagazine.com

Welcome to the October 2017 issue of TBI HOPE Magazine!

We are very pleased to present a very special issue of TBI HOPE Magazine to you this month. Over the past year, we have reached out to our readers asking a simple question: *How has technology made your life easier since brain injury?*

As expected, our readership was full of ideas, thoughts and suggestions. We have compiled the "Best of the Best" in this month's issue.

From assistive technology and devices to apps, to the importance of social networking after brain injury, this amazing issue is 100% survivor-driven. You will even read a short piece by yours truly and learn a bit about how I live day-to-day as a brain injury survivor.

We are planning to make our Technology Issue an annual event. In fact, we are already compiling stories for our 2018 Technology Issue.

It is our heartfelt hope that you find something within these pages that can make your life just a bit easier. If you have found something to be especially helpful, I would love to hear about it. You can email me directly at david@tbihopeandinspiration.com.

Peace,

David A. Grant
Publisher

Contents

What's Inside

October 2017

"Learn from yesterday, live for today, hope for tomorrow."
~Albert Einstein

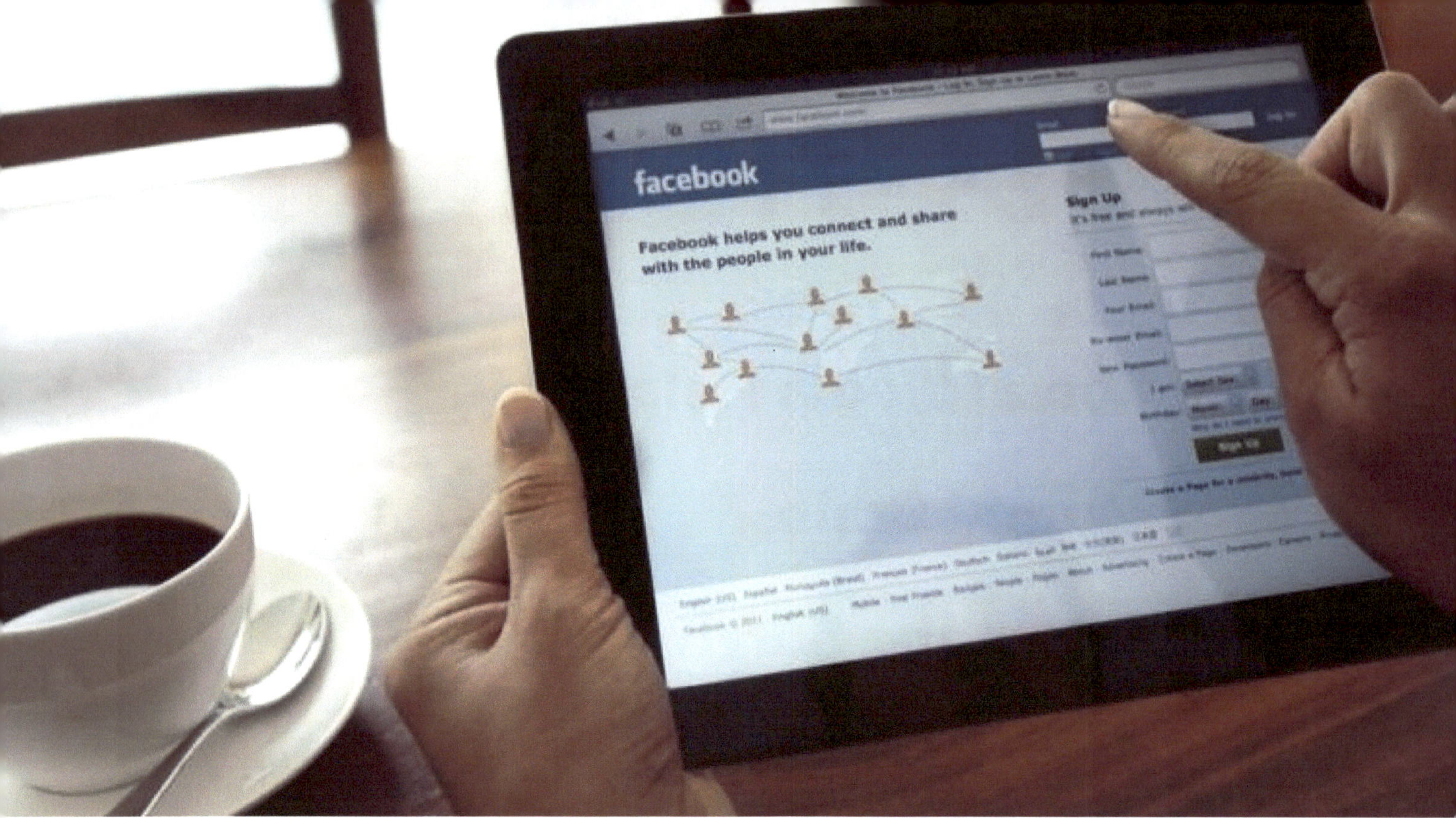

How Social Media Helped Me

By Saba Rizvi

A traumatic brain injury challenges everyday functioning. Carrying a conversation is no longer a simple task. The act of writing or speaking becomes severely difficult for those with damage to the language centers of the brain. Unfortunately, I developed aphasia, dyslexia, and other processing issues because of my TBI.

Dyslexia means one can experience difficulty reading. Sometimes the words float around on the page, while at other times they all converge together and become blurry. Sometimes, I experience a combination of the two.

Aphasia results from damage to the language centers of the brain. For some people, this means that it becomes difficult to use the correct words, or there is a mix-up of words. For example, I will say 'heat seater,' instead of 'seat heater.'

> **"Sometimes it is difficult to pronounce the correct word, as it causes physical pain in the brain."**

Sometimes it is difficult to pronounce the correct word, as it causes physical pain in the brain. It feels as if my brain wants to explode, but never gets around to it. Aphasia also contributes to difficulty reading and writing. The inability to process words, or to understand phrases and tonality is a major setback in everyday communication. You know the 'tip-of-the-tongue' phenomenon? Well, that is my every day! The social anxiety that comes along with damaged language centers is crippling. Although I have worked endlessly for years to overcome the language deficits my traumatic brain injury has caused, those deficits never go away. In fact, there are days where I see improvement, while other days are almost as bad as day one. These deficits cause severe anxiety when I communicate with people, whether in person or writing. To others, however, it is not as noticeable.

They think I am speaking or processing at a reasonable pace until the conversation comes to a halt. For me, however, I am well aware of the differences between the old me and the new me. The constant comparison of who you were before, and who you are now, never ends, despite having come to terms with it. It causes intense anxiety, which never goes away. One just learns to mask it. Just a little over a year ago, I turned to social media to express myself and share my paintings. I was forced to explain what my paintings were about, and why I created them. This meant having to overcome my language challenges and learning to be okay with the fact that sometimes I cannot adequately convey my message, or that there would be a lot of grammatical mistakes - something I was meticulous about pre-TBI.

Furthermore, an online presence meant that there would have to be everyday interaction with people. It also meant that I would have to be reading and responding constantly. This was, and still is extremely difficult, as sometimes my dyslexia and aphasia are really bad, and sometimes I can't read what is on the page in front of me. The use of social media was initially quite daunting and overwhelming, but I found it to be a great crutch over the years.

> **Just a little over a year ago, I turned to social media to express myself and share my paintings.**

There were days where I would post something, and then just avoid looking at the comments or responding for days. The mere act of posting was exhausting and overwhelming. To be able to communicate back and forth was just another battle on its own. It took me years to find a method that works for me and my disability, and even then there are still a lot of bad days. However, finding techniques has significantly helped me deal with the language disability caused by my TBI. I have found

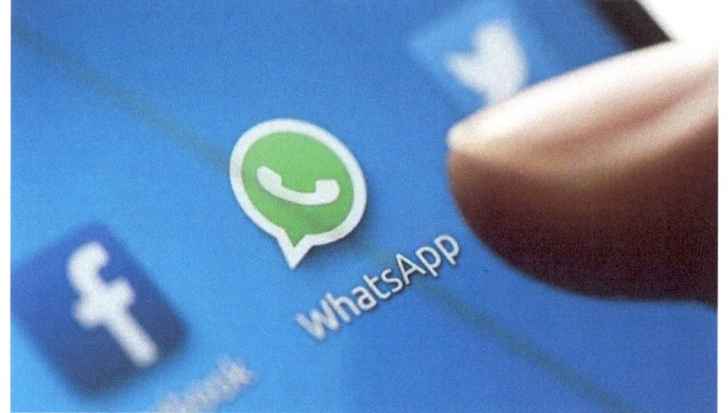

that by using social media, I can respond at my own pace, versus having to have an immediate conversation when face-to-face, or when using instant messaging apps such as 'WhatsApp.' It also means that I have the liberty to check spelling or look up definitions whenever my brain cannot process what I am trying to say. More often than not, this is the case with some everyday words, such as, 'dyslexia' or 'donut.' I can use a word every day, and then one day, it does not make any sense. Sometimes the spelling just does not seem right, or I know what the word means, but cannot find the phrase to explain what it means. The freedom to pace myself on social media has taught me that it is okay not to be able to retrieve the correct words immediately and to need more time.

Furthermore, as social media translates into real life interactions, whether it be art shows or references to posts, I am forced to overcome my momentary anxiety. The real-life interactions tied to social media generally are more 'aggressive.' They require more information recall and longer conversations. I cannot interrupt someone to inform them that I need a mental break, as that is not how discussions happen. I am frequently challenged by these interactions to carry on a conversation, to process the words and tonality, and to be able to pay attention without getting overwhelmed. As social media forces me to communicate with others at all times and on various topics, it has decreased my overall social anxiety. There are still times where my anxiety is crippling, but I focus on the times that I have overcome it.

It helps me ground myself and allows me to be patient with my deficits. The difference from a year ago to now is quantifiable, and that change in itself is motivation to keep going.

Meet Saba Rizvi

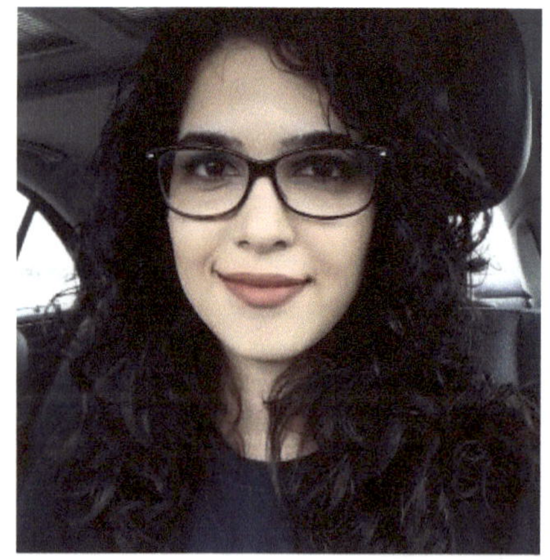

Saba Rizvi completed her HBSc. in Psychology and Exceptionality & Giftedness at the University of Toronto, and completed two years of her Doctor of Medicine. During her second year of medical school, Saba met with a horrific car accident, in which she sustained a traumatic brain injury, along with other injuries. She turned to art as a form of self-expression and therapy. Saba has exhibited her artwork at The Toronto Brain Injury Society Expressive Art Show, and the Shades of Ability Art Exhibit and Sale presented by Spinal Cord Injury Ontario. She has been featured in Eastern Eye newspaper in the UK.

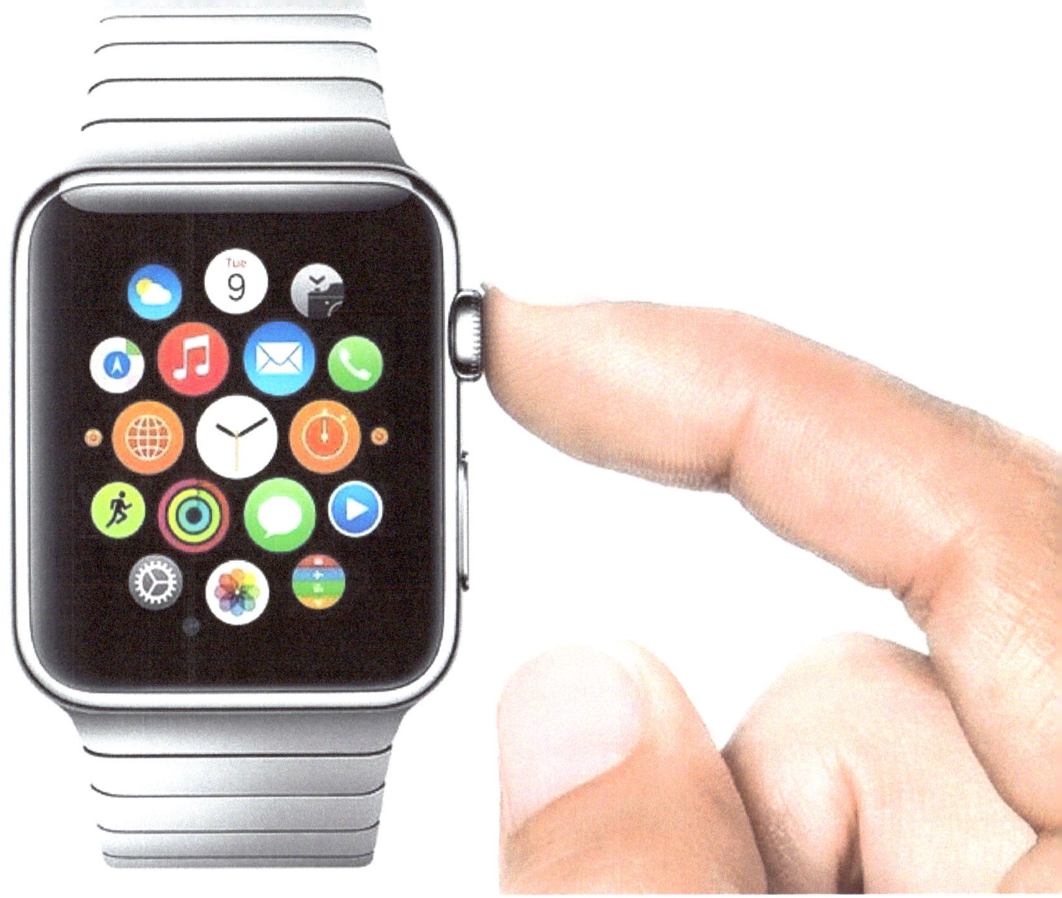

My External Brain
By Derek O'Brien

As an individual living with a spinal cord injury and a traumatic brain injury, assistive technology is essential to my independence. My iPhone wakes me up. My iPad organizes my emails, schedules, and reminders. My iWatch is a constant companion to keep my day on track. These devices are my network and my external brain. With all devices synced, the reminders are in surround sound – a song of reminders in perfect pitch.

I have been fortunate to have the opportunity to both learn how to use my technology to its fullest and to help others to learn their technology. After sustaining my brain injury, I returned to college to study New Media. This field is very technology driven. Therefore, technology became a part of every aspect of my education and daily life. Being surrounded by fellow New Media students (who were also very tech-savvy), provided me answers to any questions I had and allowed me to become proficient in the use of my devices.

> **"Since my accident in 2005, the advancements of technology have been exponential."**

Since my accident in 2005, the advancements of technology have been exponential. When I got my first power chair, it was what we consider "stock," which consisted of the basic necessities. At the time I received the chair, it suited my needs. As time went on and technology advanced even further that chair no longer suited my needs. When it came time to start the process of getting a new chair, there were features that I found out about which I needed to have implemented in my new chair. These features included a USB charger, a cell phone holder, lights, and an elevator lift. Not all of these features were available when I received my first power chair. It gives me high hopes of what the power chairs of the future will include.

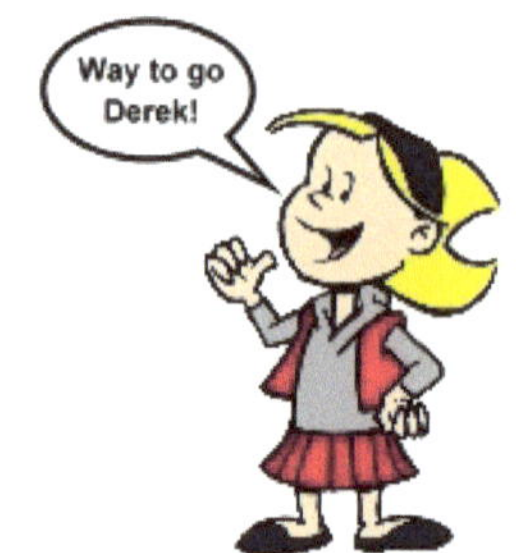

As I write this, I am awaiting my new MacBook Pro, which will further my use of technology and bring a central hub for all of my technology. The MacBook Pro can compare to your brain. Your devices are the nerves that run off of your brain. As we know with TBI and spinal cord injuries, you have to have a working brain to make your limbs work to their fullest capabilities. In today's world, the advances in technology are coming at a rapid pace. What is new today will be old tomorrow. I am very hopeful for what the future holds in technology. I continue to use my technology on a daily basis to accomplish my set goals. I look to the horizon for the next wave of technology to achieve goals I have yet to establish.

Meet Derek O'Brien

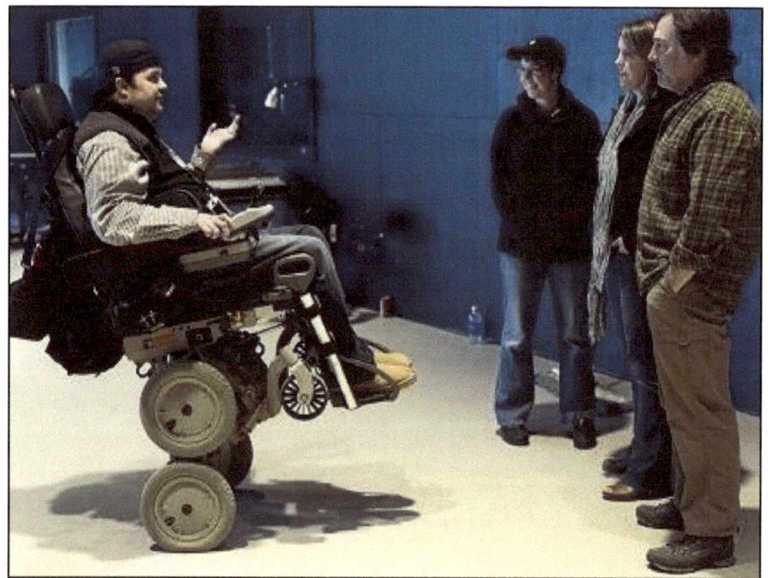

Derek O'Brien (Photo: 2102 Ungava Bay)

Derek O'Brien is a quadriplegic with a traumatic brain injury. He resides in Portland, Maine in his own apartment. Prior to his injury, Derek was studying architecture in Washington D.C. After his injury, Derek moved back to Maine, where he completed intensive therapy and ultimately returned to school. Derek is active in his community. He utilizes his degree with a job in media, and is on the board of Alpha One – Southern Maine's Independent Living Center. Derek is also a certified peer mentor for the Christopher and Dana Reeve Foundation.

Where there is no struggle, there is no strength.

~Oprah Winfrey

TBI HOPE MAGAZINE
TEST DRIVE

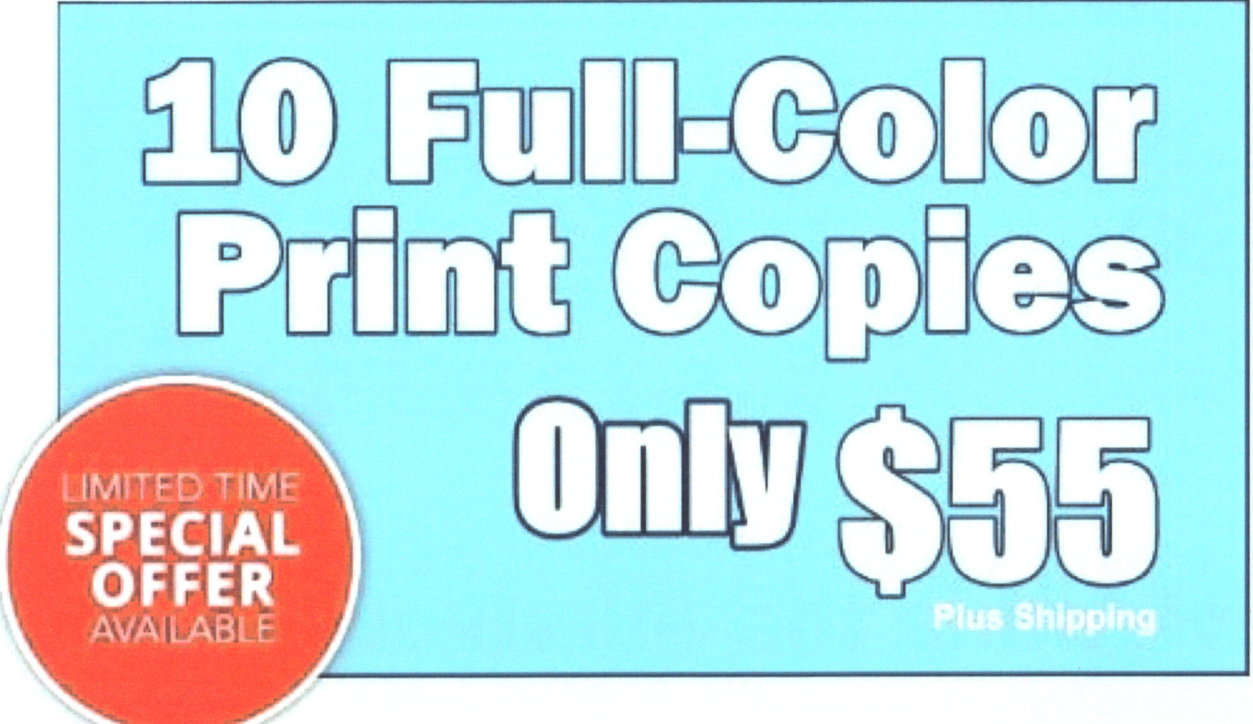

A Perfect Companion for your Support Group or Organization's Resource Library!

For More Information

Call 603-898-4540 or email info@tbihopeandinspiration.com

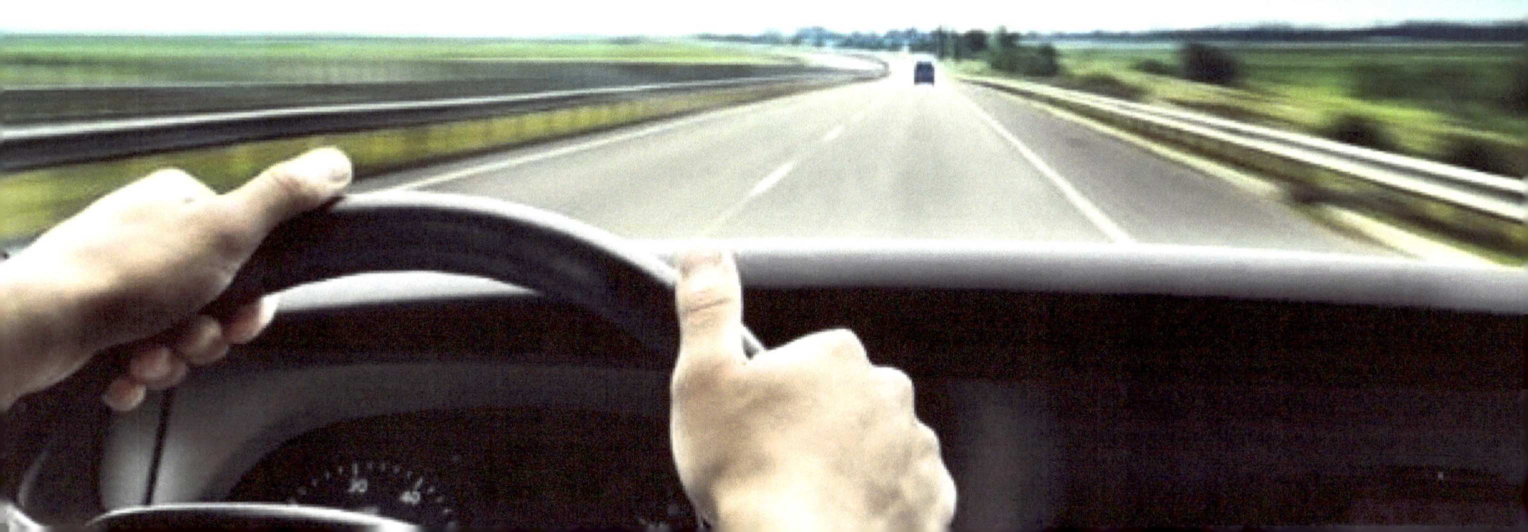

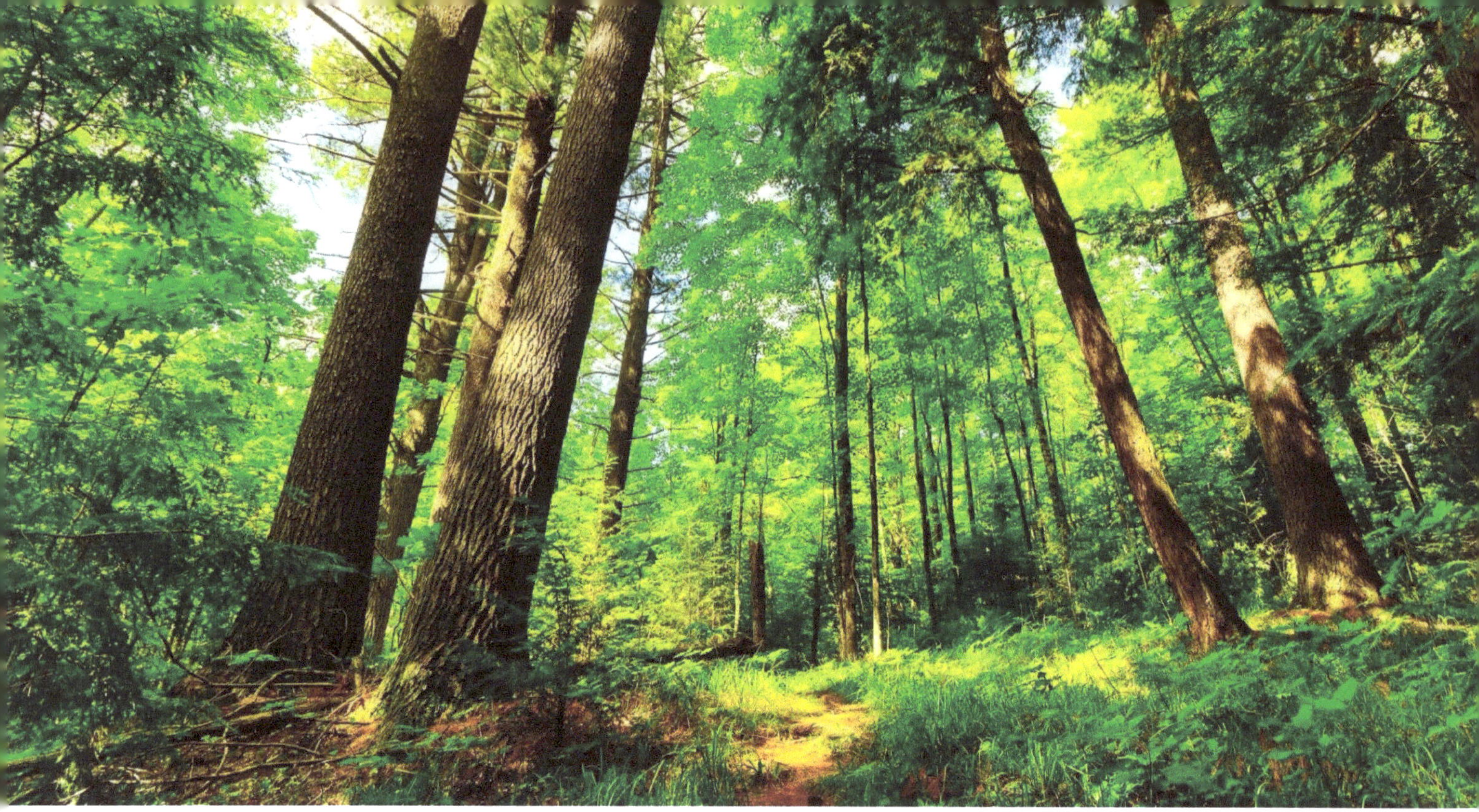

Navigating the Survivor Forest

By Pamela Donahoe

Almost three years ago, I had just finished my second year of law school, had landed a judicial clerkship, and was set on my career path. That was until I was struck by a drunk driver and sustained a bilateral subarachnoid hemorrhage. In the blink of an eye, it was all gone. I tried to go to classes, but everyone's words just sounded like gibberish. I tried to read. I recognized the words, but there was no meaning to them any longer.

I could not remember the first of the paragraph by the time I read the last of the paragraph. When I spoke, the wrong words came out or no words at all because I could not find the word I needed. When I tried to write, it was like someone else's handwriting on the paper. It did not even look like mine, and I had a tough time reading what the squiggles meant. My limitations really set in the day I tried to tell my daughter that she looked beautiful, but instead, the words "the dishwasher is purple" came out! I just broke into tears.

That was a long time ago.

> "I could not remember the first of the paragraph by the time I read the last of the paragraph."

I never was sent to any form of therapy by any of my team of doctors. Nothing! So I had to navigate the TBI Survivor forest with the most amazing and supportive family at my side. Things have come together a little for me. I can read and write better and have a little better memory. My speech has improved as well as my verbal recall. Still, I have to stop myself sometimes when the jibberish comes out, instead of meaningful words. My biggest hurdle has been my memory and executive function skills.

I tried various forms of technology, but my short-term memory was so short that as soon as I turned off alarms, I didn't even remember that the signal meant something. So that didn't work. I tried books with brain games in them but did not have the recall to complete any of the challenges. I played matching games with cards when no one was around, but never finished even once.

Then one day, my husband showed me a game on his phone called Ramsay Dash. Well, I am an avid cook and Gordon Ramsay fan, so I was ready for the challenge! I began playing. At first, it was effortless. You have to cook one thing that requires only one step. Then it builds from there. More dishes, more steps, more complicated recipes, more episodes, more challenges - and the tasks are timed. (Not only is your memory working, but it is learning to work at a faster pace.)

As you advance, you have more steps to do within shorter periods.

YOU HAVE TO REMEMBER THE STEPS ON HOW TO PREPARE THE DISHES!

However, don't worry, if you forget, the game has a way for Gordon to show you again. I found my saving grace.

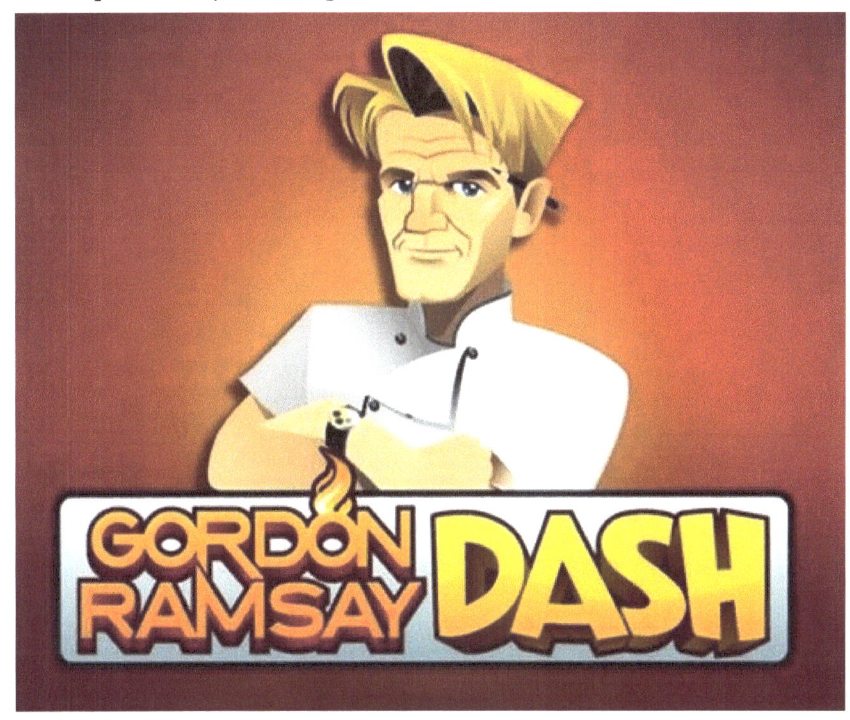

I played the game day in and day out. I opened every restaurant one at a time and achieved every goal the game offered. Slowly, my memory began to improve. Not just within the app, but in my day-to-day life.

Today, I still play the game religiously, several episodes a day. I still use my whiteboard to remind me of conversations I have had with my husband in which we set boundaries for our kids. I have a calendar on my kitchen counter that I look at every morning to let me know what I have scheduled that day. I use sticky notes for everything. Before bed, I have my family text me things they need me to handle the next day, but I do not open the text. That way, when I turn on my phone in the morning, I see unopened text messages, read them, and complete the tasks. They are there in writing, just in case I need to refer back to them. In addition, I have an office, a space dedicated to me away from the rest of the house, where I will not be distracted. It is my happy place. My office is where I go to organize my life. It might take hours of sitting at my desk, or just minutes, to figure out what needs to be done and when, but it is my special place to go and work it out, no matter how long that might take.

I am thankful for the Ramsay Dash game because, without it, I would not have the memory function that I do have; albeit not perfect, it surely is better than it was before Ramsay Dash. So, no matter how silly something may seem, be willing to try. You never know what will trigger your memory to work again. In addition, I am learning that survivors know much more about managing life after TBI than doctors ever will - I rely on them for nothing. My family and I have read, studied, looked for sources and case studies, talked this through over and over and what we have found on our own has been astounding. Never give up hope on this long and lonely journey. The tiny milestones will come - slowly, but they WILL come.

Meet Pamela Donahoe

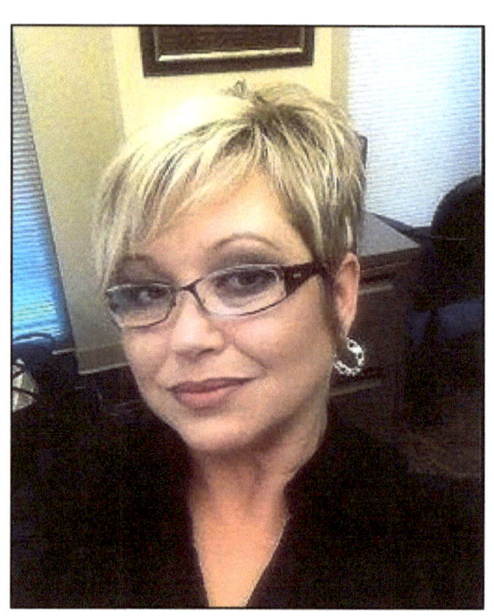

Pamela is a TBI Survivor. Prior to being hit by a drunk driver, she had a career in State Government and was seeking her Juris Doctorate so she could practice law. Now disabled and having never received therapy, she searches for ways to navigate the TBI experience.

She is married to her high school sweetheart, love of her life, TBI caregiver, and best friend, Ronnie Donahoe. They have three children, Amanda, Dakota, and Riley, who are adults. Together with her family, they wish to share their story.

"It always seems impossible, until it gets done."

~Nelson Mandela

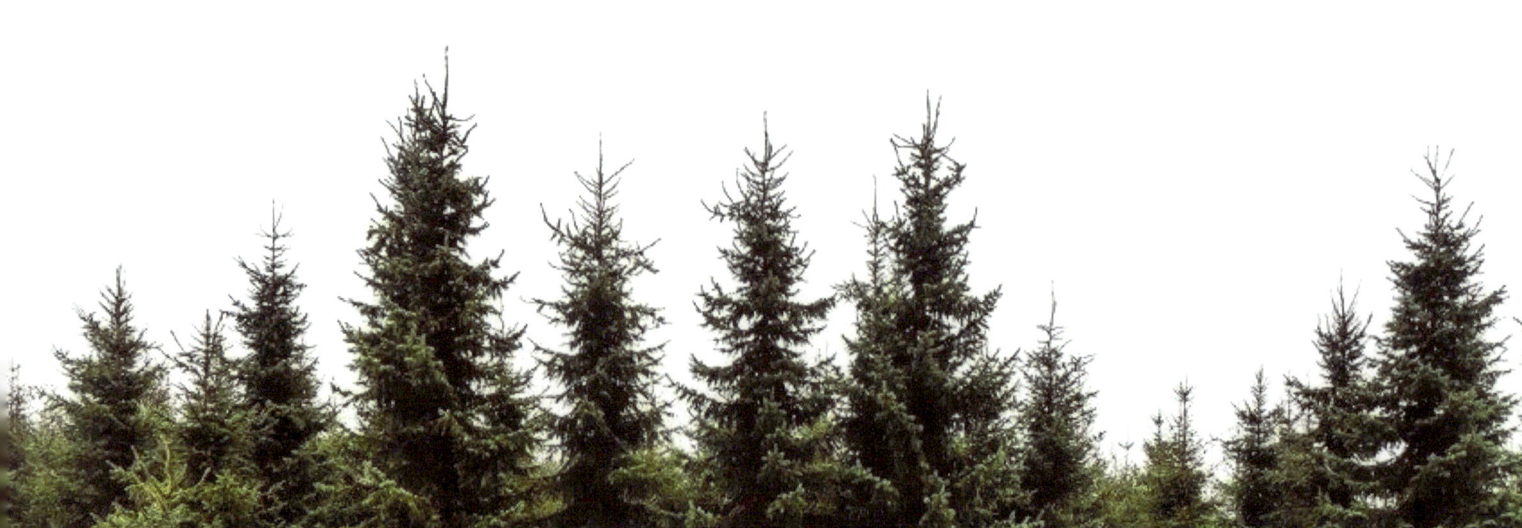

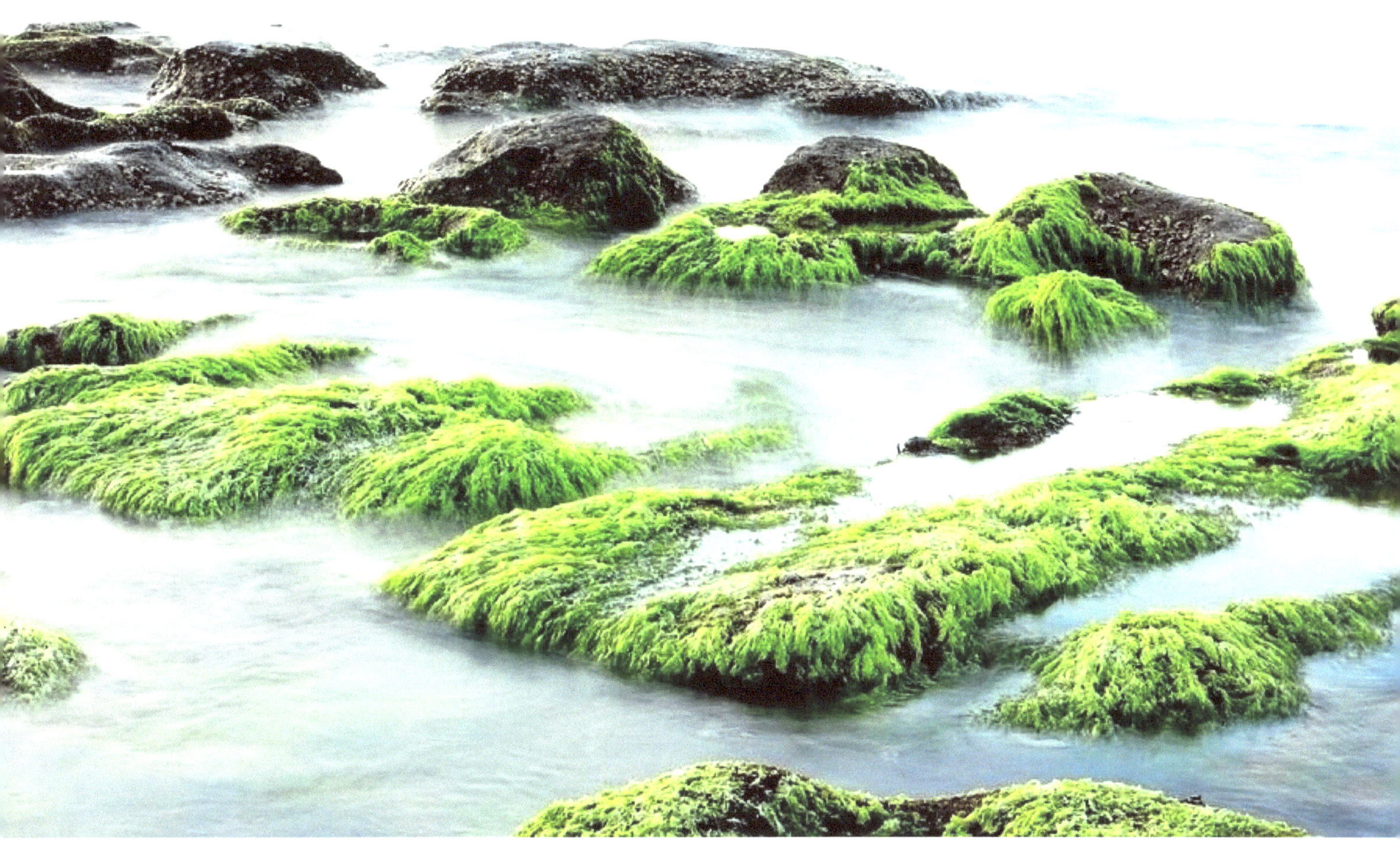

How Seaweed Might Heal Brain Injury

By Arlene Weintraub

Traumatic brain injury (TBI) causes long-term irreversible damage largely because inflammation prevents the regrowth of healthy brain tissue. So Australian scientists went on the hunt for a natural compound that could halt that inflammation—and they found it in something that's plentiful in their country: seaweed.

Scientists at Australian National University and RMIT Australia University worked with Tasmania-based biotech company Marinova to develop a compound derived from a sugar molecule in seaweed. They combined the substance with short peptides and created a brain scaffold, according to a press release. The scaffold closely resembles healthy brain tissue.

 In the lab, they injected the mixture into a damaged brain. The scaffold prevented scarring and improved healing. And it seemed to have a positive effect on brain cells located far from the original injury site. They published their findings in two papers, in the journals Nature Scientific Reports and ACS Biomaterials Science and Engineering.

"This potentially allows an entirely natural, biomaterial approach to treat the damage caused by traumatic brain injury and stroke by allowing the brain to repair itself," said Richard Williams, a senior lecturer at RMIT, in the release.

Tamping down inflammation after TBI is a major focus of researchers around the world. Last year, scientists at Hebrew University in Israel announced they were testing a molecule that targets the inflammatory protein thioredoxin (Trx1) in mild brain injury. And the University of Miami partnered with Tetra Discovery to test an experimental drug that may enhance memory formation in neurons following brain injury.

The Australian scientists believe that their seaweed-based hydrogel changes how the brain reacts to injury, allowing it to regenerate when it might not have otherwise. They plan to explore whether the material can be applied to repairing bones, muscles and nerves.

Article Reprinted with permission by Arlene Weintraub and FierceBiotech.

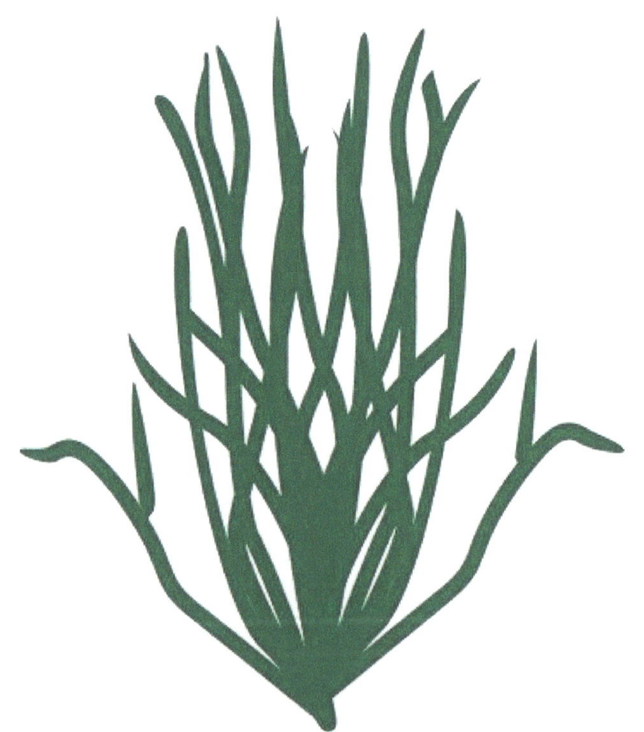

Meet Arlene Weintraub

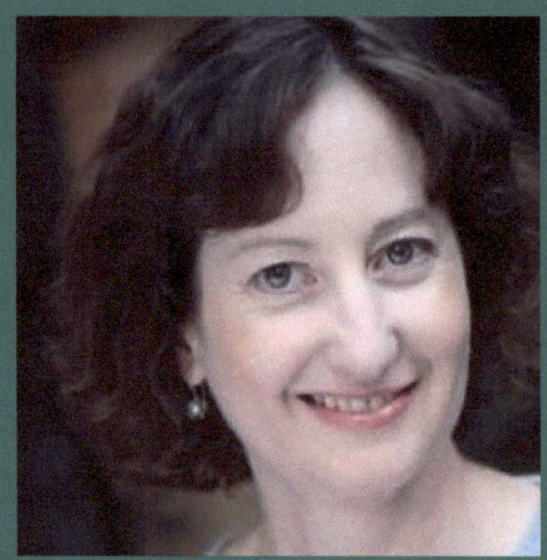

Arlene Weintraub has over 15 years of experience writing about health care, pharmaceuticals and biotechnology. Her freelance pieces have been published in the New York Times, US News & World Report, Technology Review, Scientific American, USA Today, Entrepreneur.com, FierceMarkets and other media outlets. She was previously a senior health writer for BusinessWeek, covering both the science and business of health.

She also worked as an editor for Xconomy.com, covering the biotech industry, as well as technology, life sciences and clean technology companies. She has won awards from the New York Press Club, the Association of Health Care Journalists, the Foundation for Biomedical Research, and the American Society of Business Publication Editors.

Her book about the antiaging industry, Selling the Fountain of Youth, was published by Basic Books in 2010.

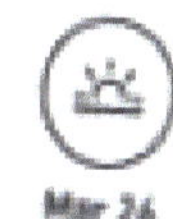
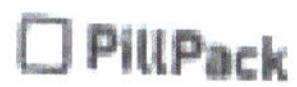
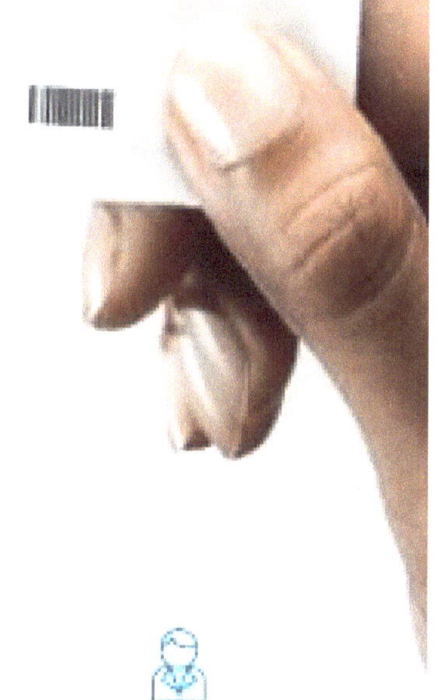

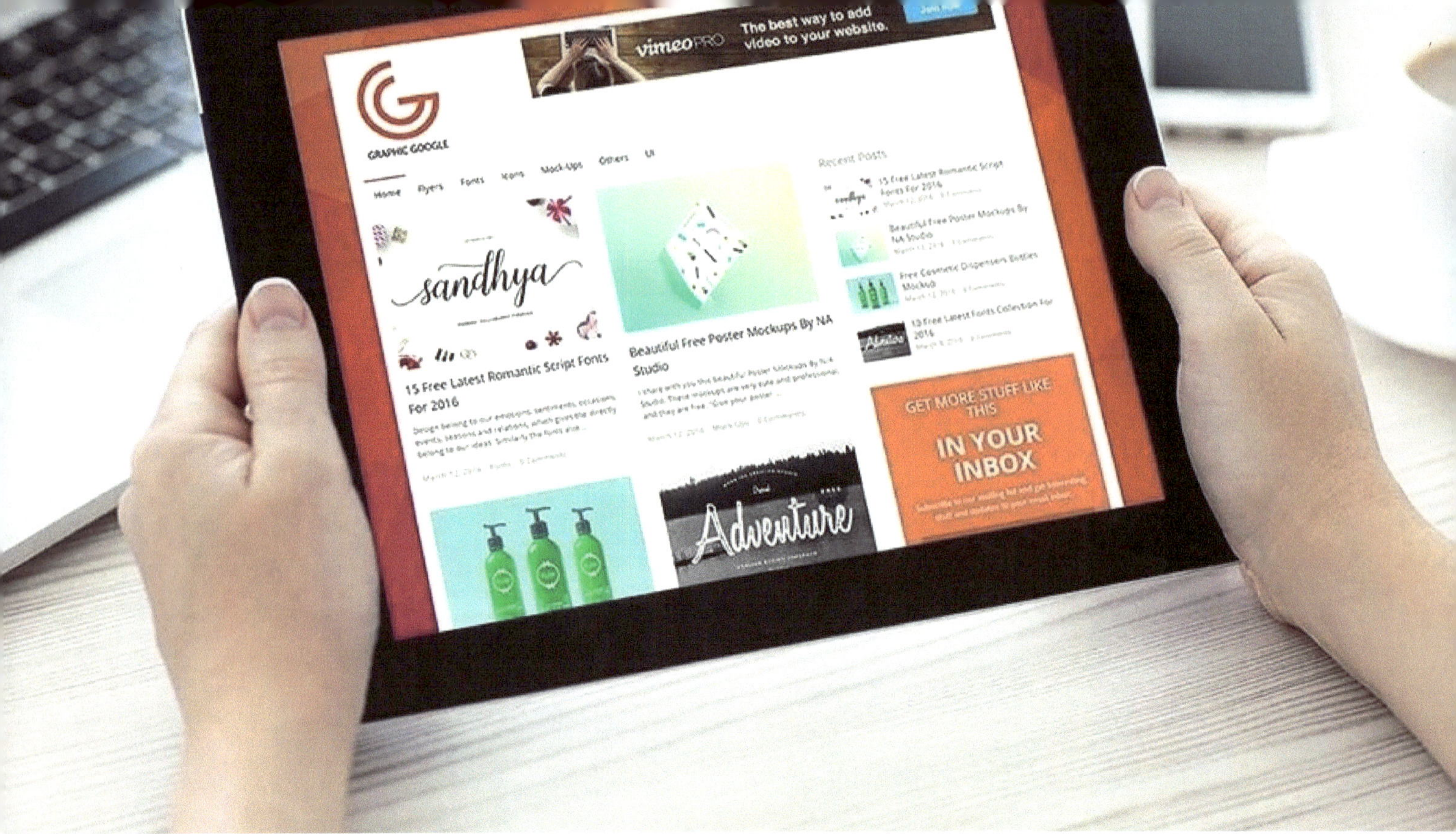

How Technology Helped Me

By Jennifer Stokley

I was so lost for the first five years after my brain injury, like being caught in an ever-present fog. I fought hard and finally found my way out, slowly. A few moments, then an hour or so at a time (now five years later, I'm out mostly all day, every day). Back then, any time out of the fog was better than none. Everything was so confusing and new. I had to relearn everything in the short times that I was out of the fog.

I had to learn when to take my necessary medications and make sure I did not take more than prescribed, from forgetting I had already taken them (short-term memory loss issues!) I had a friend program alarms on my "smartphone."

If I was busy, in the middle of something and could not stop and take my medications right away, I was able to push one button that put the alarm on "snooze," and it would go off again in a little while to remind me.

"I had to relearn everything in the short times that I was out of the fog"

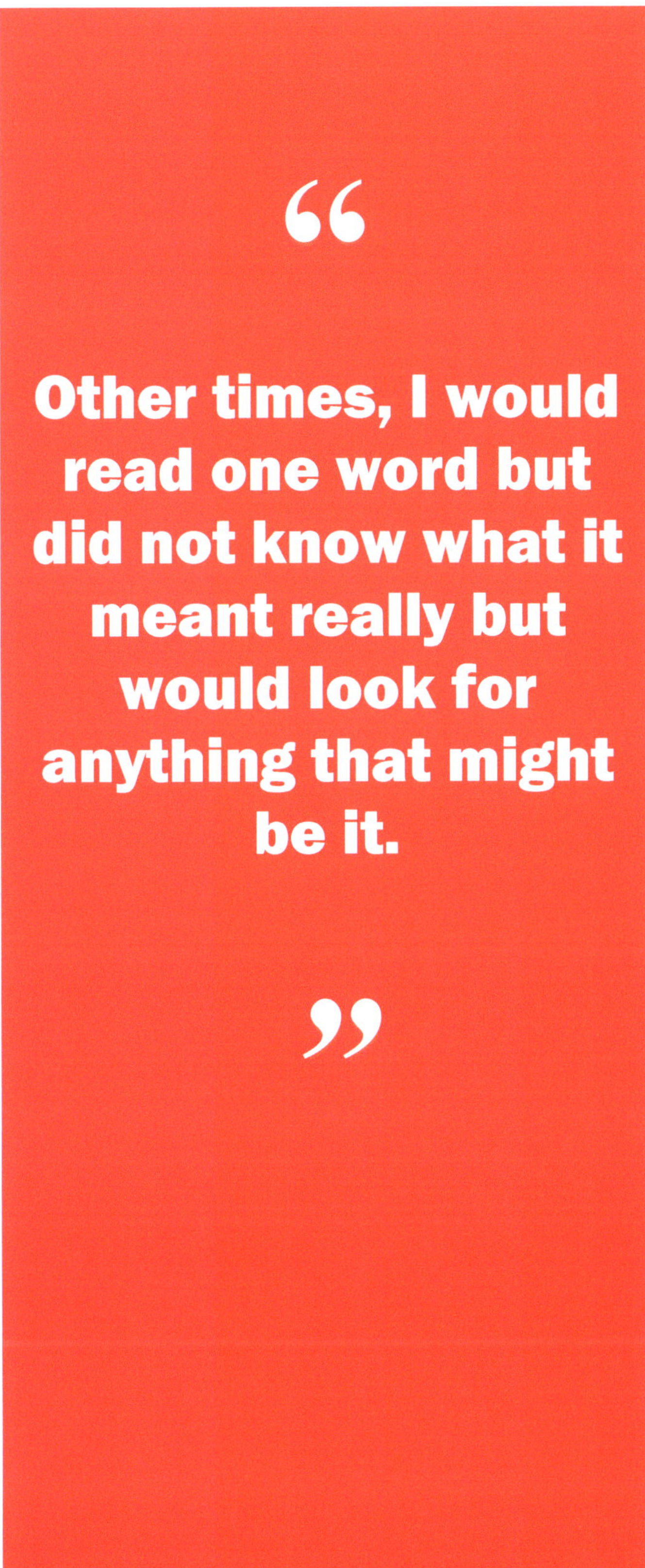

Once I took my pills, I could forget them. If no alarm sounded, I did not have to think about my medications at all. What a huge relief! Living alone, taking too much is a serious issue for many, by accident, with short-term memory loss!

Then I had a family member send me an iPad. It was neat, but I had no clue what to use it for at first. Then I found a Hidden Object Game on my regular computer and had a friend add it to my iPad. I began very, very slowly. It had words to read, then a picture of lots of stuff to look through to find the things with the phrase. Often I would read one word, be looking and looking, get frustrated and look at the word again and realize I read the wrong word!

Other times, I would read one word but did not know what it meant really but would look for anything that might be it. I found if I said the word aloud first, then began looking, I did so much better. There was also a puzzle of the picture that I had to put back together. In addition, there was a speed bonus where I had to read the words, find the pictures, and get as many as possible in a certain amount of time.

This game, I have been playing for over four years now. I take a break every hour or so, relax and forget about everything for a couple of minutes, and just focus on the game itself. I now rarely read words wrong,

I rarely have problems finding the objects, my speed has increased, my speech is much better, and I am much better at the puzzles and visual things in general.

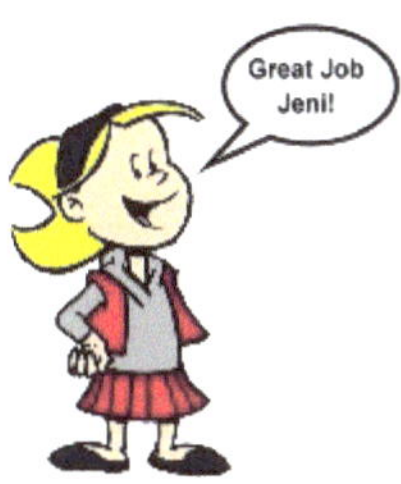

Overall, this has helped me cognitively in more ways than I could explain. I am more alert to things around me; I read much better now, I know the meaning of more words, I can speak better from saying the phrase aloud, etc.

These two technical devices have helped my recovery process in so many ways; one gave me independence and safety, the other gave me cognitive training and more!

Meet Jennifer Stokley

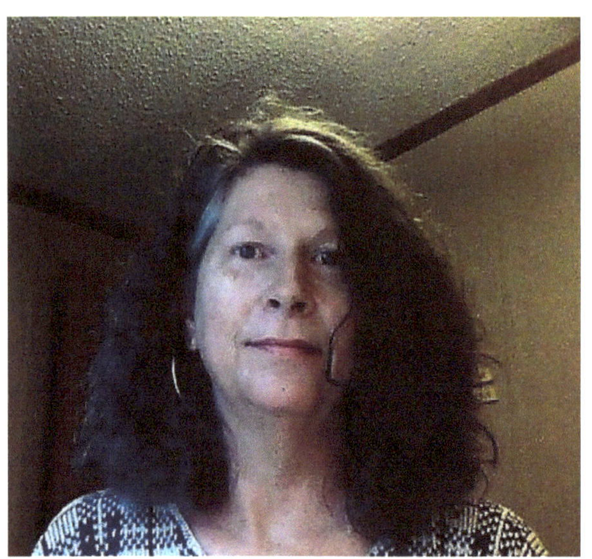

Meet Jeni. She had her TBI in May of 2007. She fell out her second floor window to the sidewalk below. Jeni broke her neck, five ribs, her pelvis in three places, ruptured her bladder, punctured her lung, went into Cardiac Arrest twice and incurred a brain injury. She was in a coma for three weeks, then a rehab hospital for two months. Jeni lost forty-two years' worth of pre-TBI memories. "I'm not going backwards anyway, I'm only living for today and working towards tomorrow and beyond," shares Jeni. "The past is gone, tomorrow is never promised, all we truly have is today. Make the best today we can. That's all that truly matters!"

Living With Hope

By Patrick Brigham

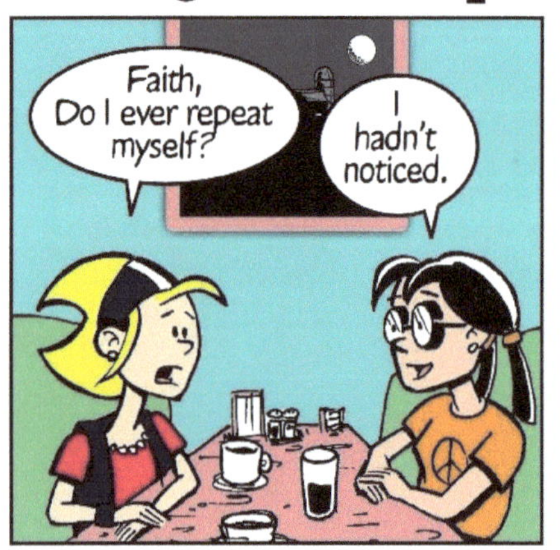

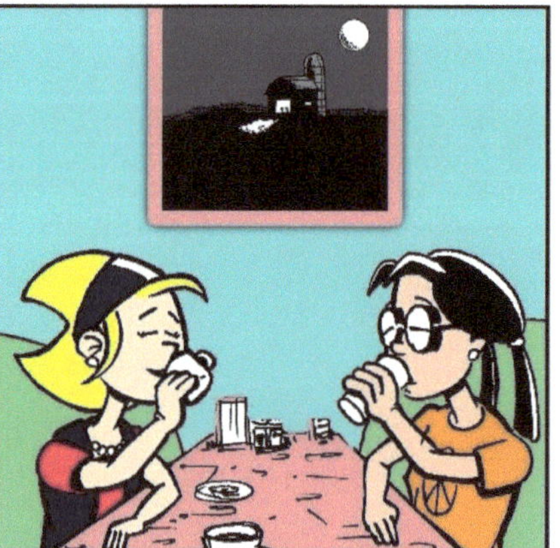

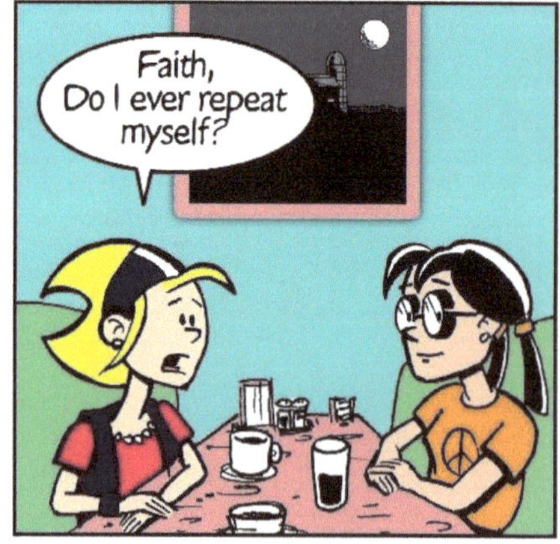

Navigating a TBI with GPS

By Tristan Greenman

It is 9:30 PM and I find myself driving around the neighborhood again, looking for my husband. He went outside to feed the dog thirty minutes ago and did not come back in. He is nowhere around our house. It is dark; the bugs are out, it's cooling off.

It is 10:30 AM, I am at work, and one of my husband's caregivers calls me to let me know Tim is missing. He had one of his fits, stomped off into the woods, and is nowhere to be found.

There are tracking systems for cars; law enforcement uses them to locate stolen vehicles. Rental agencies and car dealerships use them for lease cars. There are tracking systems for phones and pet collars. You can find out where your kids are by pinging their phones, and you can locate your furry family members too. But how do you track a TBI patient who suffers memory loss and has bouts of deep confusion? How about some GPS shoes!

My husband, Tim, suffered a TBI from a motorcycle accident when a utility truck ran a stop sign. He is nothing short of a miracle in his recovery efforts. Physically he has healed, but his TBI leaves him mentally unprepared for continuing his life as it was before the accident.

> **"How do you track a TBI patient who suffers memory loss and has bouts of deep confusion?"**

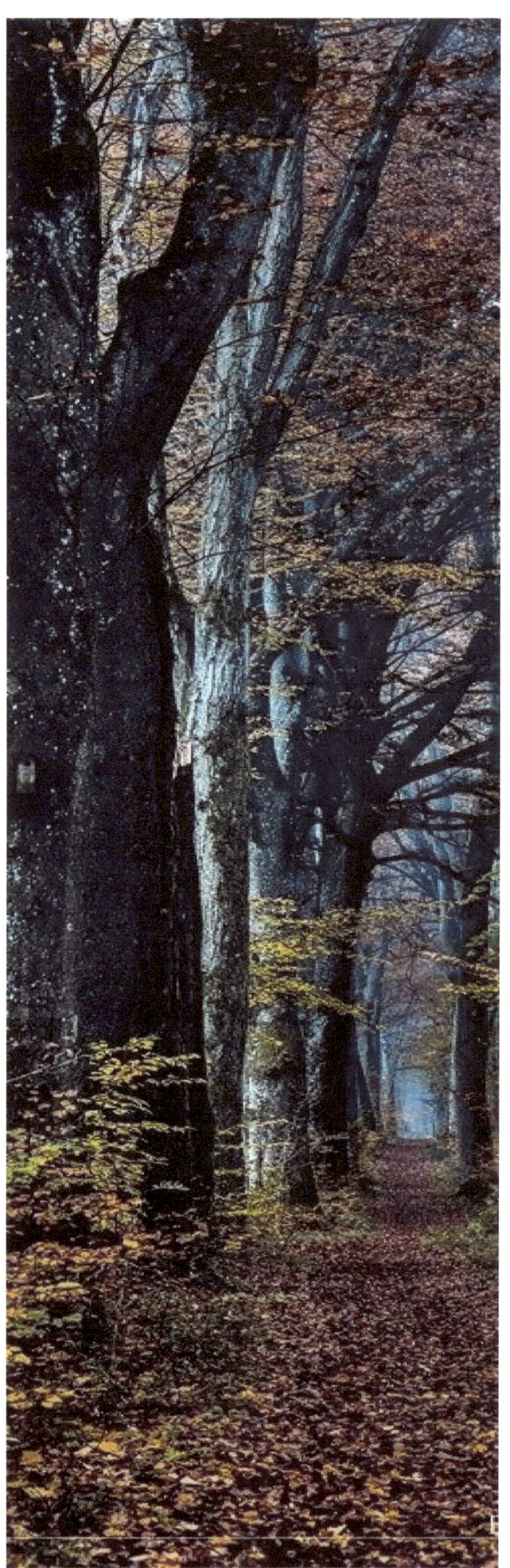

He cannot drive. He cannot remember to carry a phone, and I tried to modify a dog-tracking collar to fit onto his belt, but it was cumbersome and foreign to him, so he ditched it. Tim loves to be in the woods, but has become lost several times and ended up far from home and exhausted.

His exhaustion adds to his confusion, and only the grace of living in a safe community who keeps tabs on him has brought him back safely. He usually drives a golf cart around the neighborhood and visits a circuit of seniors, but often forgets he has a cart and walks around aimlessly, again confused about where he is and where he should go.

Enter GPS shoes. Actually, these are not shoes; they are insoles hidden inside his shoes, so he does not have to remember to carry anything. They are based on smartphone technology and linked to an app on my phone. They come in a couple of different sizes and can be trimmed to fit one's shoes. I found these on the internet, advertised for Alzheimer's patients and autistic persons.

For a monthly fee, the peace of mind I get from being able to find him when he wanders off is worth it. As well as the sense of independence he gets from not having me fuss around his ramblings. He comes and goes, many times without telling me that he is off to see so and so, and rather than panicking, I call up my app and find out just where in the neighborhood he has gone.

There has only been one instance of him trekking off without his shoes on, and he did not get far before the discomfort of the terrain on his feet forced him back to the house. These insoles have to be charged like a phone and are comfortable for him to wear. I do not think he remembers they are in his shoes.

I struggled with whether or not to begin tracking him, but in one of his more lucid moments, Tim told me that I should do whatever I needed to do to feel better about our situation. Well, I feel more than better. I feel like another weight has lifted from my shoulders.

I cannot limit his mobility; he has always been a get-up-and-go person. After breaking 37 bones in his body, healing, and physical therapy, I don't WANT to limit his mobility. Get up, get out, and do something has been a mantra around our house - just be careful.

These insoles do not help the memory loss or confusion that resulted from Tim's TBI, but they are as helpful to me as any medical treatment or therapist we have been to in the past four years. I let him go, and then pull out my phone and go with him.

Meet Tristan Greenman

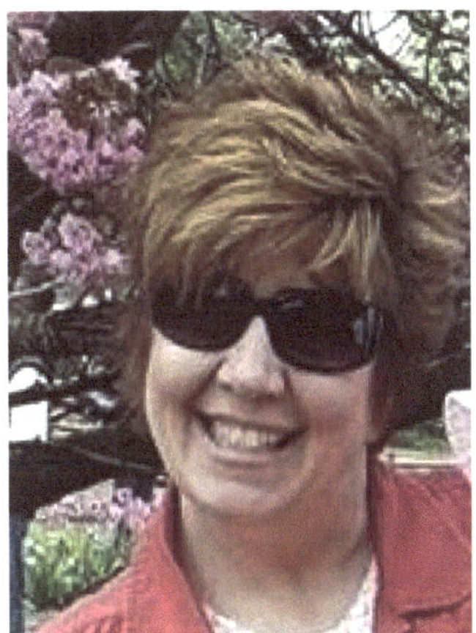

Tris is caregiver to her husband, Tim, in Southwest Michigan. She also works full-time as an accountant and tries to keep their lives on an even keel and regular schedule.

She and her husband enjoy fishing, gardening and spending time with the grandbabies. "TBI has taught me to have infinite patience and to appreciate friends and the therapy community so much more!"

> # "The one who falls and gets up is stronger than the one who never tried."
>
> **~Roy T. Bennett**

Join our Facebook Family

What do over 25,000 people from over 40 countries and five continents all have in common? They are all members of our vibrant Facebook family at /TBIHopeandInspiration

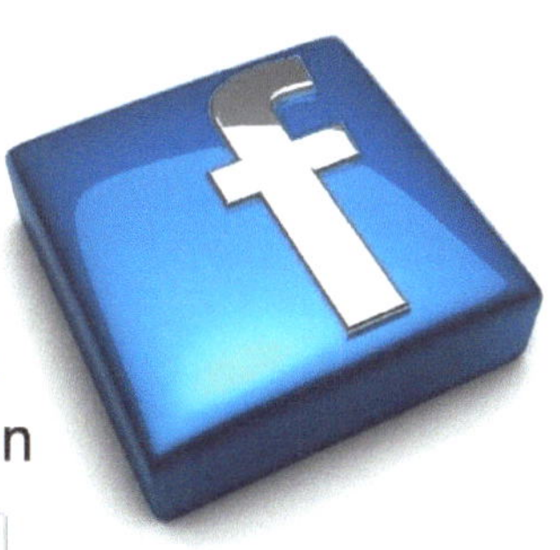

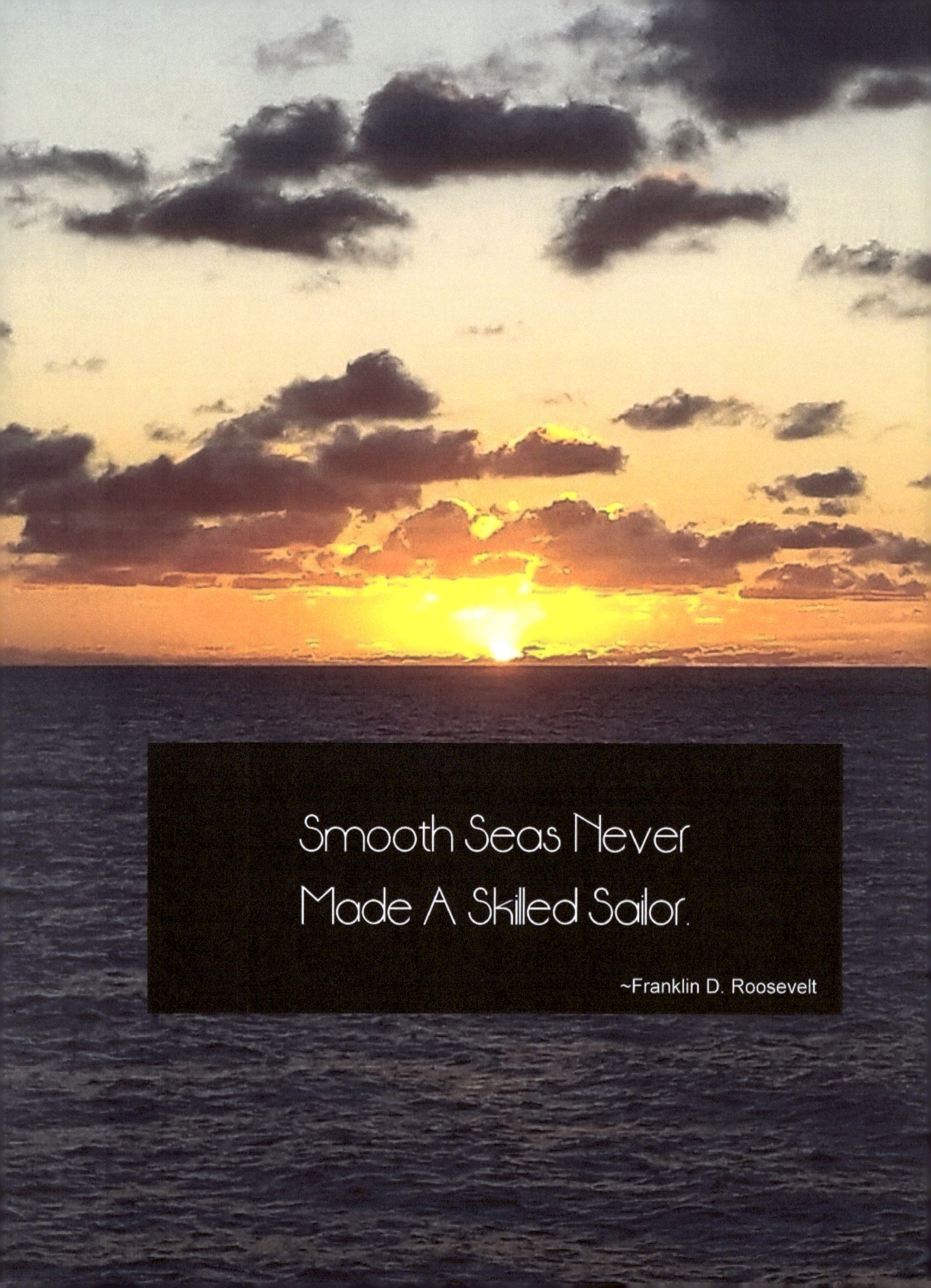
Smooth Seas Never
Made A Skilled Sailor.

~Franklin D. Roosevelt

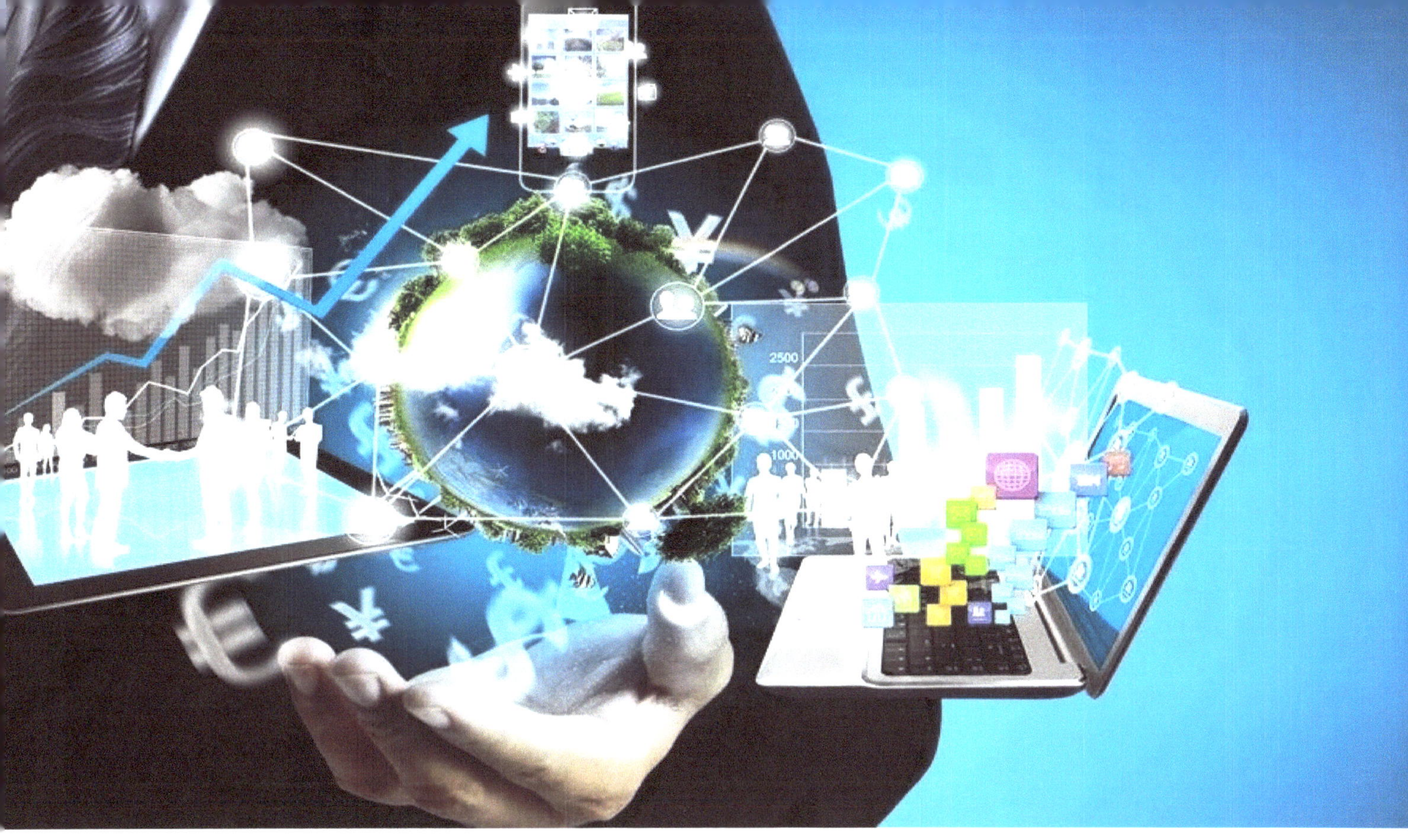

My Tech-Driven Life

By David A. Grant

For many years, I was a quintessential multi-tasker. I ran my own successful marketing company, fielded calls from clients all day, answered emails, and was adept at staying on top of the day-to-day tasks required to run a bustling and thriving business.

All of that came to a screeching halt in late 2010 when I was struck by a car. My injuries were life changing and included broken bones, torn ligaments, and a traumatic brain injury. Life as I knew it was about to get tough.

During the first few months after my injury, it became apparent that my memory was severely compromised. I was unable to tell the day of the week, what month we were in, or even the year. My daily life, which had been smooth and relatively trouble-free, was becoming problematic.

> **"During the first few months after my injury, it became apparent that my memory was severely compromised."**

Knowing that memory issues were a challenge, I decided to try sticky notes. I am a product of the Technology Age, so I decided to use digital sticky notes on my computer. I found a PC app that let me pick the note color, and inscribe notes as needed. There was even a handwriting-like font, making it feel like real sticky notes.

For a few weeks, I made a note of this, crafted a reminder for that, and moved forward writing sticky note after sticky note. There was one problem though. While I was good at writing notes, I completely forgot to read any of them. Six months or so later, I accidentally stumbled upon my note folder and saw a long list of uncompleted tasks. And so ended that experiment.

Over the ensuing years, I occasionally tried technology to help me navigate the not-so-subtle nuances of my life as a brain injury survivor. Nothing lasted for long. But over time, for every few tech-tricks I tried, one would stick.

Keeping appointments and remembering important dates was an ongoing problem. I wished one of my sons a happy birthday a day late. If I could have a dollar for every missed call or appointment I experienced early on, I'd have enough money for a nice night out with my wife, Sarah. As a Google user, I started to use the Google Calendar feature. I entered just about everything into my calendar. Kid's birthdays, so easily remembered before, were added to my calendar. My wedding anniversary, my parent's birthdays, and their wedding anniversary were entered. If it was an important date, it made it to my Google calendar.

It took me a couple of years, a couple of complete calendar cycles, to get all the important dates covered. Here is where it gets fun – my Google calendar syncs with my cell phone and my tablet.

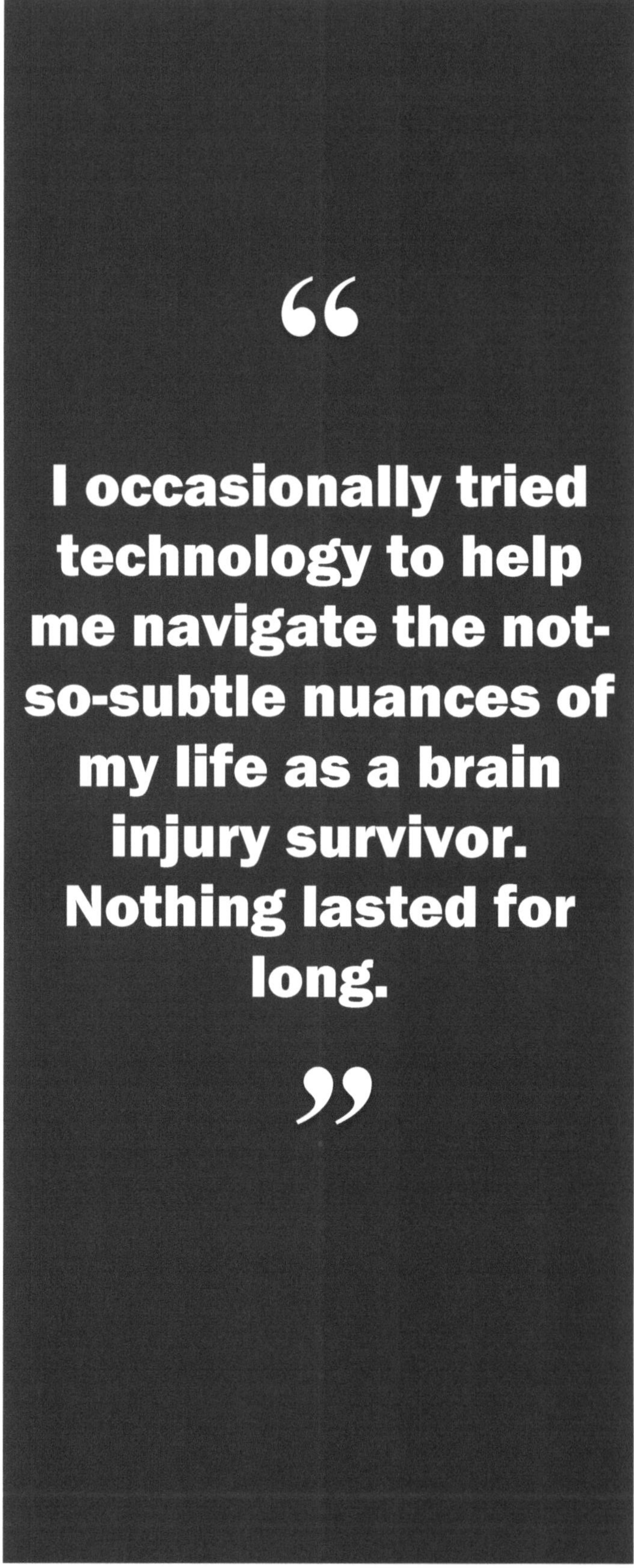

As I set reminders for most anything of importance, pretty much every device I have lights up with reminders. This "in your face" method works well for me. In fact, it's impossible to miss.

Sometimes, over the course of a phone call, a friend might mention an upcoming birthday. As I now habitually note dates, I will enter the event into my calendar – and promptly forget that it's there. A year later, I get the reminder. When I reach out to wish someone an entirely unexpected "happy birthday," I am always met with surprise. "You remembered!"

Yeah, you could say that.

It creates the appearance of memory and means that important tasks, dates or anniversaries are no longer missed. It has been a game-changer for me. Unlike my early sticky note experiment, I don't need to remember to read my notes. In many respects, I am now more efficient than I was in my pre-injury life. But my love-affair with tech doesn't end there.

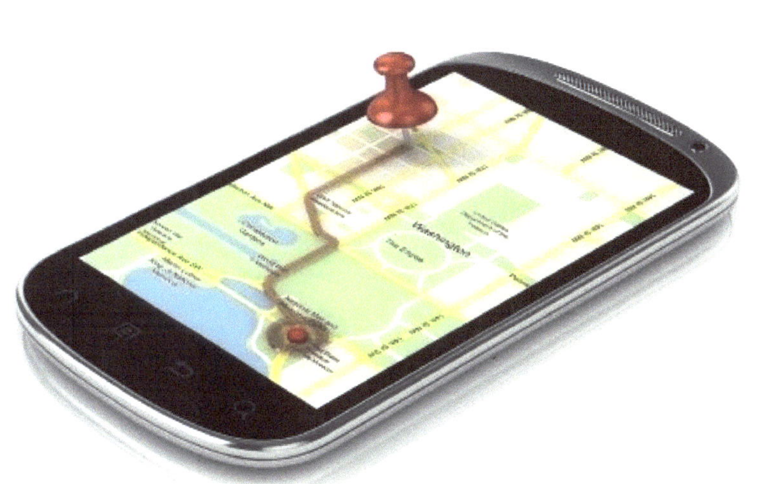

My cell phone has become a lifesaver for me in many ways. In addition to living with a brain injury, I am also a diabetic. Taking my medications on time and as directed keeps me healthy. These days, I use a medication tracker app called MediSafe. It lets me input my daily medications and reminds me when it is time to take my medication. It is easy to use. Better still, it's a free app. Either missing my medication or double-dosing my medications can be dangerous. When my phone reminds me that it is time, it's time. Along the same lines, I use an app to monitor my blood sugar.

Sure, having diabetes is not a brain injury challenge, but like many people, I have health issues beyond my brain injury. Apps like these simplify my life and help keep me on track for total wellness.

These days, my wife Sarah and I are out and about, living life. We have both come to depend on technology in other ways. Getting from Point A to Point B used to be easy. But seasonal challenges here in New Hampshire include jaw-dropping traffic jams during some of our peak seasons. Pulling out my phone, I can say, "Okay Google, Driving directions to _______________." I'll let you fill in the blank. These days, Google uses dynamic routing to get you around and offers options that circumvent traffic jams. As a brain injury survivor who is fortunate enough to drive, traffic jams can steal my mental energy fast, leaving me wiped out for the rest of the day – or even the rest of the week. Problem solved!

Of course, we use apps like All Trails to find quiet places to walk; Trip Advisor helps when we are not close to our neighborhood, as well as a few other apps that simplify life.

Our newest foray into tech is our new assistant Google Home. Like the Amazon Echo, this is an artificial intelligence device now in our living room. I can ask Google what I have on my calendar for the day, how heavy traffic is, how warm the day will be, etc. I can even request it to play my favorite music. We are a month or so into the Google Home experience, but almost daily I find new ways for this device to assist me as I navigate today's ever-complicated world.

Everyone has his or her own journey, a path to follow as unique as the individual does. What works for me might not be the best fit for someone else, but I encourage you to try tech as a way to compensate for what you might have lost. You have nothing to lose, and perhaps a simpler life to gain!

Meet David A. Grant

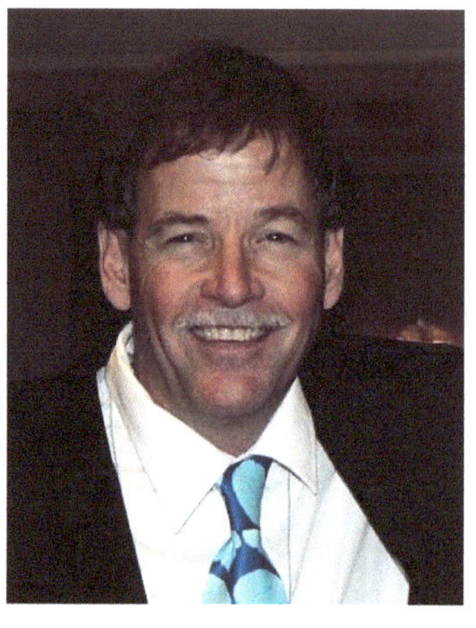

David A. Grant is a freelance writer based out of southern New Hampshire and the publisher of TBI HOPE Magazine. He is the author of Metamorphosis, Surviving Brain Injury.

He is also a contributing author to Chicken Soup for the Soul, Recovering from Traumatic Brain Injuries. David is a BIANH Board Member as well as a member of the Brain Energy Support Team Board of Directors. David is a regular contributing writer to Brainline.org, a PBS sponsored website.

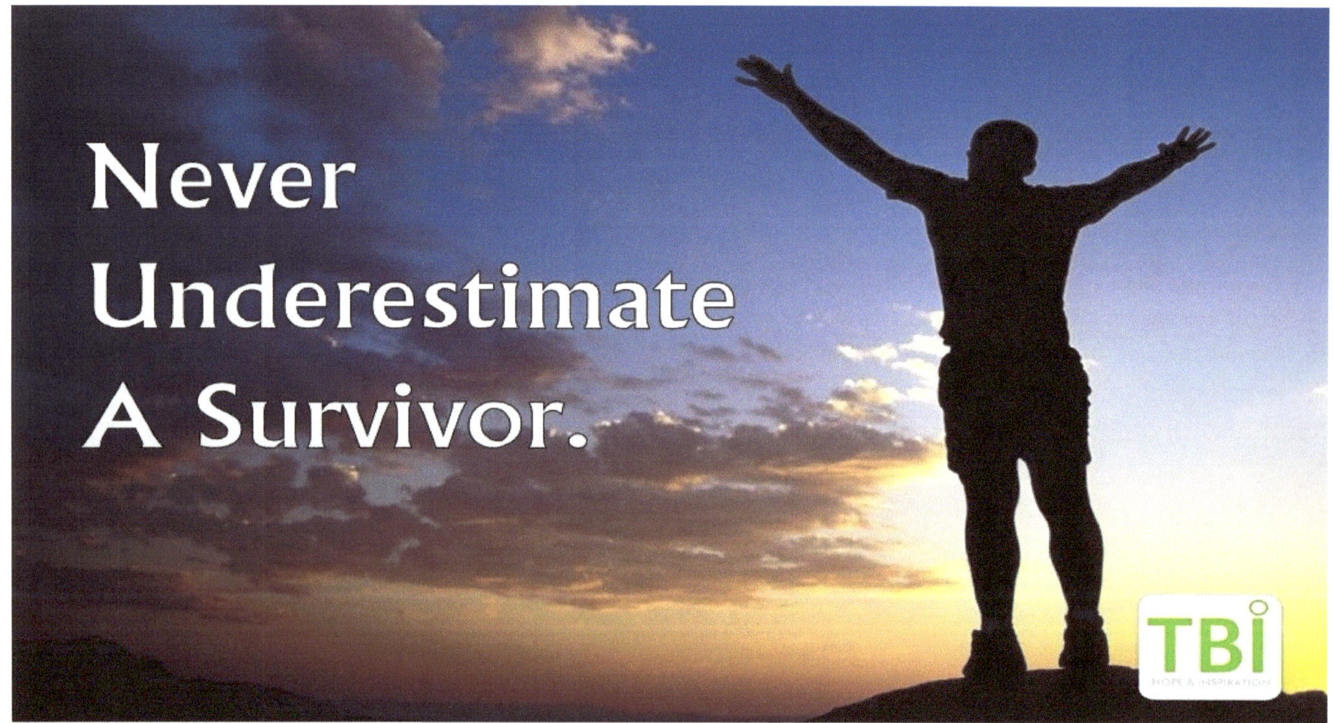

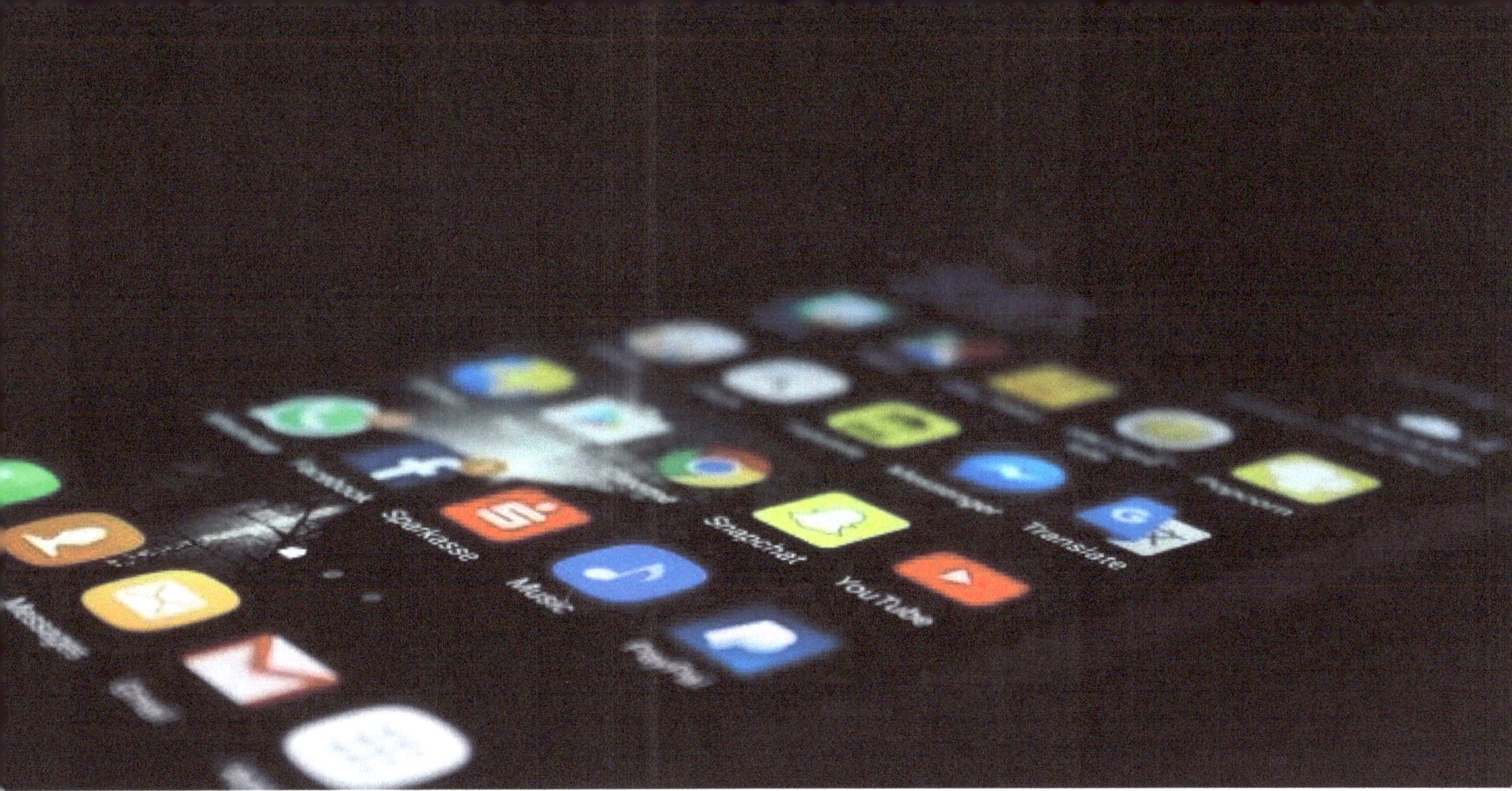

Life-Changing Mobile Apps
For People with Brain Injury

Almost every day, we hear of new mobile device applications ("apps") developed for just about everything — from staying organized to finding pharmacies or restaurants while on the road. It's hard to keep up.

The BrainLine team sorted through many resources to compile this list of apps for mobile devices for people with a brain injury, their families and caregivers.

Some of these apps have proven to be especially helpful for people with brain injury. The phone can be used to remind you of an upcoming appointment or to take medication, or it can be used like a traditional paper notebook to keep all your addresses, telephone numbers, calendar items, lists, and ideas. Please note that BrainLine does not endorse these or any specific products.

Many of these apps are free, while others are paid apps. Check the Google Play Store or iTunes Store for current pricing and availability.

Audible - Listen to books on your mobile device. Great for people who have trouble reading or who retain information more effectively by listening.

Answers:YesNo - Easy to use, affordable way for you to communicate with those around you if you are nonverbal. The app has two, large, color-coordinated buttons--one for yes, and one for no. Press either, and a voice will read you selection.

 Awesome Memory - Card game to help you improve your memory. All of the cards are laid face down on a surface and players take turns flipping two cards face up. The object of the game is to reveal pairs of matching cards. Similar to the traditional game of "concentration." * *Paid version available that includes advanced levels and functionality.*

Behavior Tracker Pro - Application that allows caregivers, behavioral therapists, aides, or teachers to track behaviors and automatically graph them. Option to record video of behaviors or interventions to later review with doctors, parents, teachers or therapists.

Breathe2Relax - Hands-on stress management tool with diaphragmatic breathing exercises. Designed to help you with mood stabilization, anger control, and anxiety management.

Clear Record Premium - Audio recording app that suppresses ambient, background noise allowing the user to record conversations in noisy environments while maintaining clear voices. Control play-speed without modifying pitch-quality. Slow down conversations to a manageable pace for the user.

Concussion Recognition & Response - Helps coaches and parents recognize whether an individual is exhibiting/reporting the signs and symptoms of a suspected concussion. In less than 5 minutes, the app allows a coach or parent to respond quickly to determine whether to remove the child from play and the need for further medical examination.

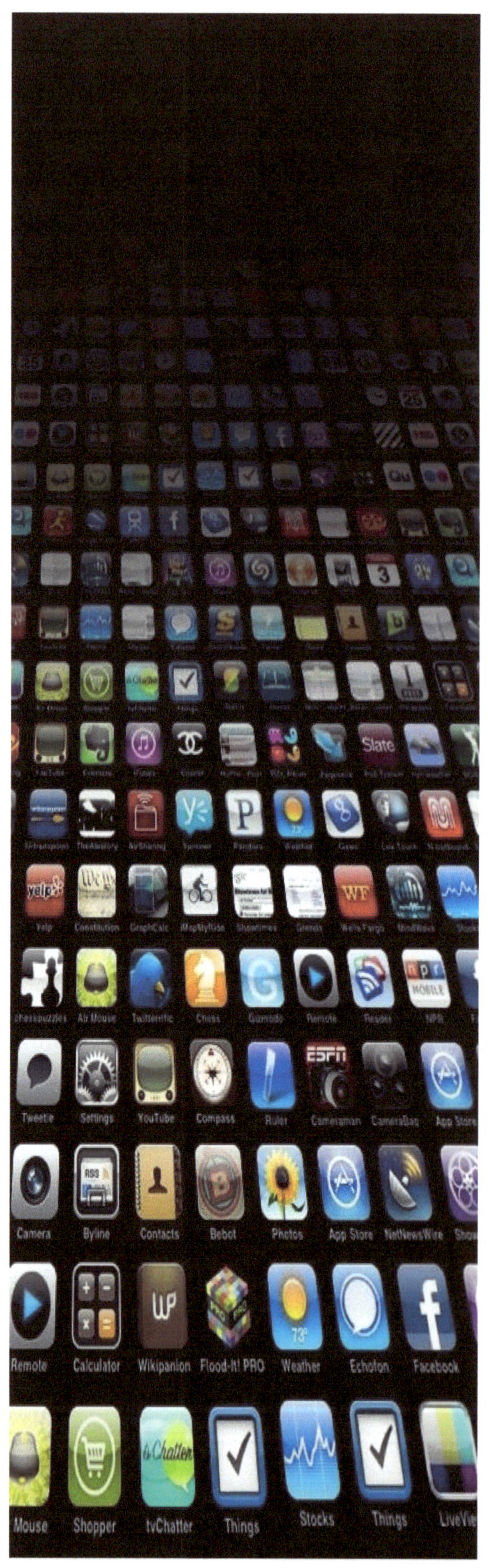

Corkulous Pro - Family life organization app that includes a shared calendar, shopping lists, to do lists, family journal. This app allows you to stay in sync with your family. ** Paid version available for advanced functionality.*

d2u Dictation and Transcription - Voice recorder with integrated transcription service* provides you with a comprehensive dictation and transcription solution. Record, edit, and upload a digital recording then have the file transcribed to text. HIPAA compliant. ** Transcriptions are a paid feature.*

DialSafe Pro - Learn proper phone usage and safety with an app that allows for hands-on practice. Learn these critical skills through the use of animated lessons, skill building games, practice sessions, and a realistic phone simulator.

Dragon Dictation - Voice recognition app that allows users to easily speak and instantly see their words on the screen. Send short text messages, longer email messages, and update your Facebook and Twitter statuses without typing a word. Help remember everything across all of the devices you use. Stay organized, save your ideas and improve productivity. Take notes, capture photos, create to-do lists, record voice reminders, and make notes completely searchable.

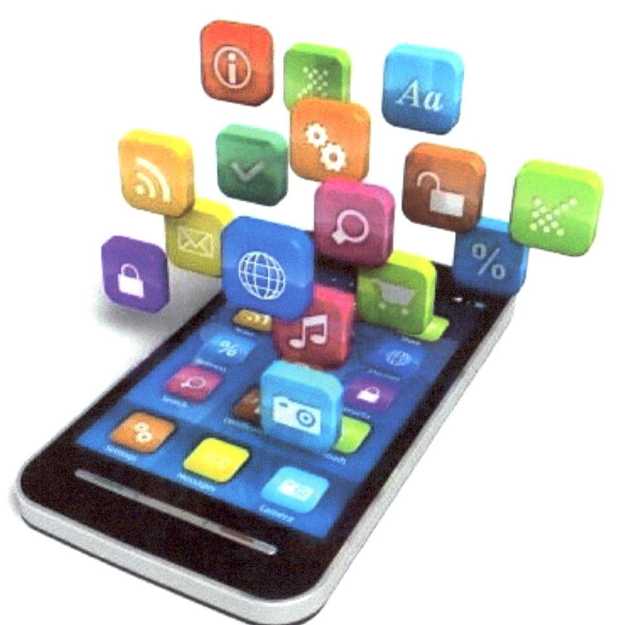

Find a Pharmacy - Immediately find the closest pharmacies to your location based on your device's location or address.

Find My iPhone - Location app for iOS that tracks wireless devices and enables a you to track where the devices are, where they have been, and enables you to send warning messages or tones to those devices.

Flashcards Deluxe - Flashcard app which can be used to study just about anything you want. Built in dictionary, capacity to include pictures and sounds, zoom into pictures, and auto-repeat sounds on the cards.

iBooks with VoiceOver - Search and instantly download thousands of popular book and magazine titles. iBooks works with VoiceOver, which will read the contents of the pages out loud.

ICE (In Case of Emergency) - Store all the information you might need in an emergency in one convenient location. Names of doctors, medications you are taking, medical conditions, allergies, and insurance information can be accessed with the tap of a finger. You can also use the app to find hospitals nearby in case of an emergency.

Index Card - Non-linear writing tool that helps capture your ideas and store notes as they come to you. Organize the flow of your thoughts by using a familiar corkboard interface and compile your work into a single document.

Lumosity - Brain exercises targeting memory, attention, speed, flexibility, and problem solving. You can design your own personalized training, including "courses" with TBI- and/or PTSD-specific content. *Paid subscription available for advanced features.*

MakeChange - This app will show you the best way to count change so that you use the least number of coins. Slide and stack coins until you have the amount shown on the register display and check your answer.

Matrix Game - Helps you develop visual perception skills such as visual discrimination. It can also help you to develop attention and concentration, spatial orientation and principles of classification and categorization. * Paid version available for advanced levels and more functionality.*

n-Back - n-Back is designed to improve your working memory through actively memorizing and recalling information.

Naming TherAppy - Handwriting app that helps you get the fast, tactile gratification of writing on paper, with digital power and flexibility. Take notes, keep sketches, or share your next breakthrough idea — in the office, on the go, or at home.

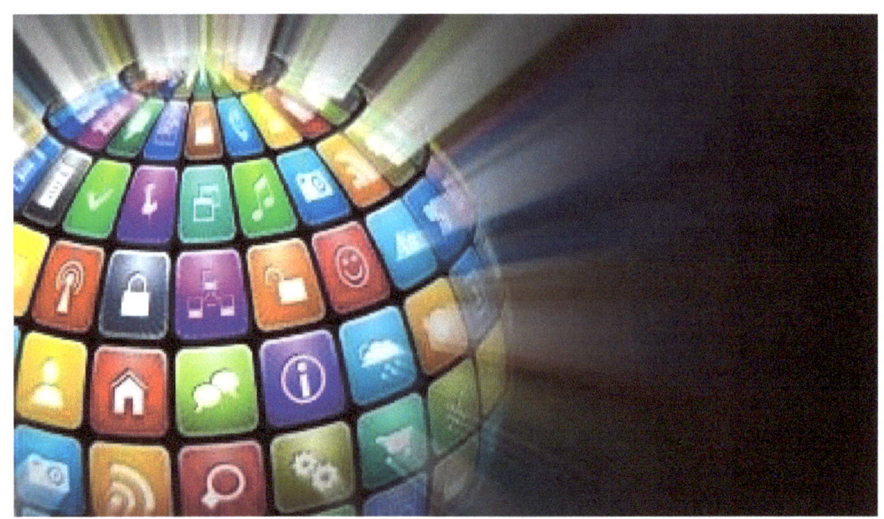

Pictello - Create visual stories and talking books. Each page in a story can contain a picture, a short video, up to ten lines of text, and a recorded sound or text-to-speech using natural sounding voices.

Pocket SCAT2 - This application is a shortened version of the SCAT2 test and is designed to be used in a field setting by coaches or parents to help identify possible concussions.

Proloquo2Go - An alternative communication solution to help you if you have difficulty speaking. Natural sounding text-to-speech voices, high-resolution, up-to-date symbols, powerful automatic conjugations, a vocabulary of more than 7,000 items, and advanced word prediction.

PTSD Coach - Designed for veterans and service members who have, or may have, post-traumatic stress disorder (PTSD). Education about PTSD, information about care, a self-assessment for PTSD, help finding support, and tools that can help you manage the stresses of daily life with PTSD.

Quick Talk AAC - This app gives a voice to those who cannot speak for themselves. Quick and flexible app designed to help you talk as quickly as possible.

SpeakWrite Recorder - Voice recorder that turns your phone into a fully functional dictation system. Record, edit, and send your audio. App integrates with SpeakWrite's 24/7 paid transcription service. Compile your dictation, upload, and within a few hours receive your transcribed document.

SoundAmp - Assistive app that turns the iPhone into an interactive hearing device. Using the microphone or a headset with a microphone, it amplifies nearby sound making it easier for you to hear.

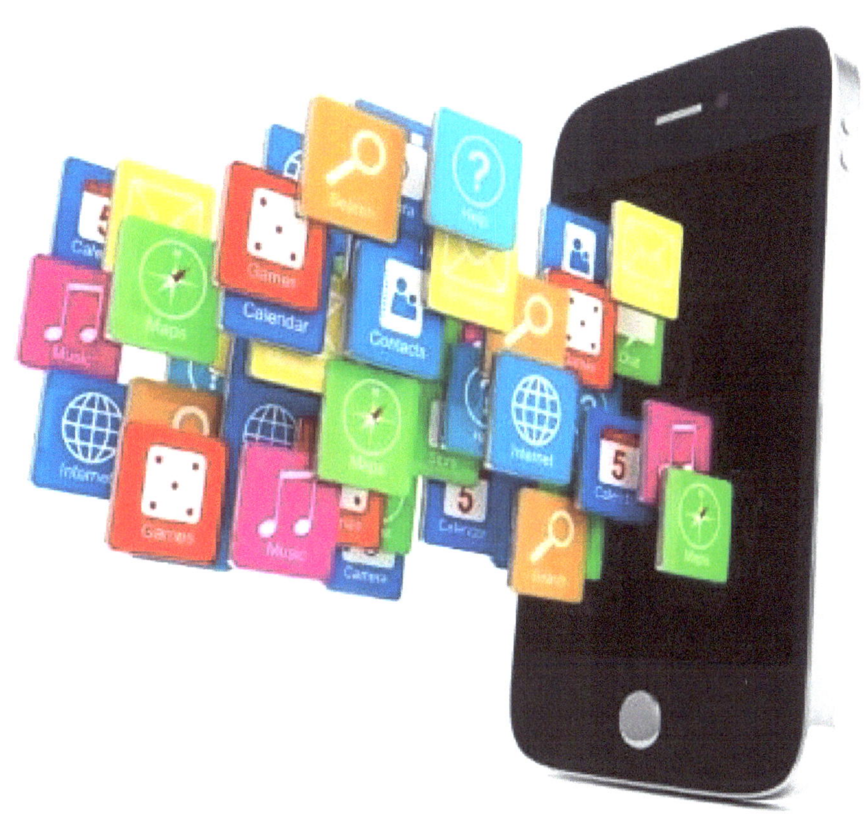

Spaced Retrieval TherAppy - Facilitates recalling an answer over expanding intervals of time (1 minute, 2 minutes, 4 minutes, 8 minutes...) helps to cement the information in memory, even for those with impaired memory.

T2 Mood Tracker - Designed for service members and veterans, this app helps you self-monitor, track, and reference emotional experiences associated with common deployment-related behavioral health issues like post-traumatic stress, brain injury, depression, and anxiety.

Tap2Talk - Alternative means of communication app. Push pictures of items to have a voice speak them for you.

TextTwist - Word game app where you try to find the word that uses all of the letters on the screen as fast as you can. Crossword mode lets you complete a crossword puzzle using a limited number of letters. Word of the Day mode offers a daily puzzle.

Today Screen - One-stop app for quickly viewing your upcoming agenda, tasks due, and your local weather forecast. Tasks and events are intuitively highlighted based on date and time, so that what you need to look at right now stands out clearly.

Touch Calendar - Touch Calendar makes viewing your calendars easy. See your whole calendar at a glance. No more flipping between different calendar views. Touch Calendar does it all from one zoomable and scrollable view. This app is especially useful for people with attention problems who do better with fewer steps.

Unus Tactus - Developed to assist people of all ages with mild cognitive and/or motor deficits by allowing you to have an easy to use cell phone, with a simple set up. It utilizes a one--touch photo dialing system to generate phone calls using phone numbers from your existing contacts or those that you import directly.

Voice4U - Picture-based, augmentative and alternative communication (AAC) application that helps you express your feelings, thoughts, actions, and needs.

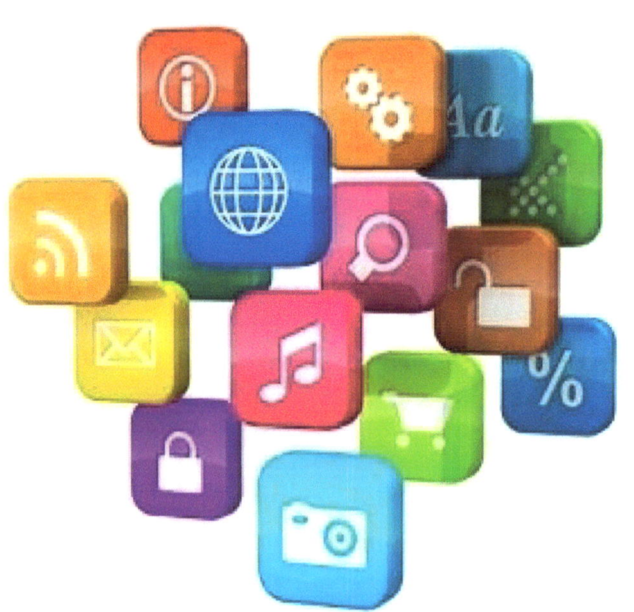

Verbally - Comprehensive Augmentative and Alternative Communication (AAC) app for the iPad. This app enables real conversation for those who have challenges speaking. Just tap in what you want to say and Verbally speaks for you. *Premium features available with an in-app purchase*

Visual Schedule Planner - Customizable visual schedule iPad app that is designed to give you an audio/visual representation of the events in your day. In addition, events that require more support can be linked to an activity schedule or video clip.

Voice Cards Are Not Flashcards - Create voice flashcards with an autoplay and shake option. Create sets of flashcards just as you would with paper flashcards, except you create a voice recording of your questions and answers in sets of Voice Cards. You can "flip" between questions and answers by swiping or shaking the phone.* *Two versions, lite with limited functionality, $0.99 for full version.*

Where Am I? - View and share your location, including your city, zip code, telephone area code, and approximate street address as well as the times of sunrise and sunset and GPS latitude and longitude.

Word Warp - Game with which you can create as many words as possible from a selection of letters. If you're stuck, just press the "warp" button and it will help you out.

Used with permission from BrainLine.org, a WETA website. www.BrainLine.org.

News & Views

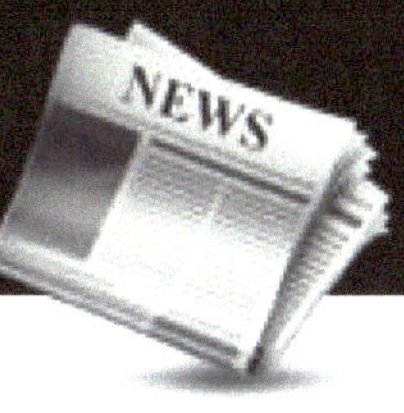

Sarah and I would like to again thank this month's contributing writers. As you have just seen, survivors are embracing today's available technology in ways that make life easier, and improve their day-to-day ability to navigate through an increasingly complex world.

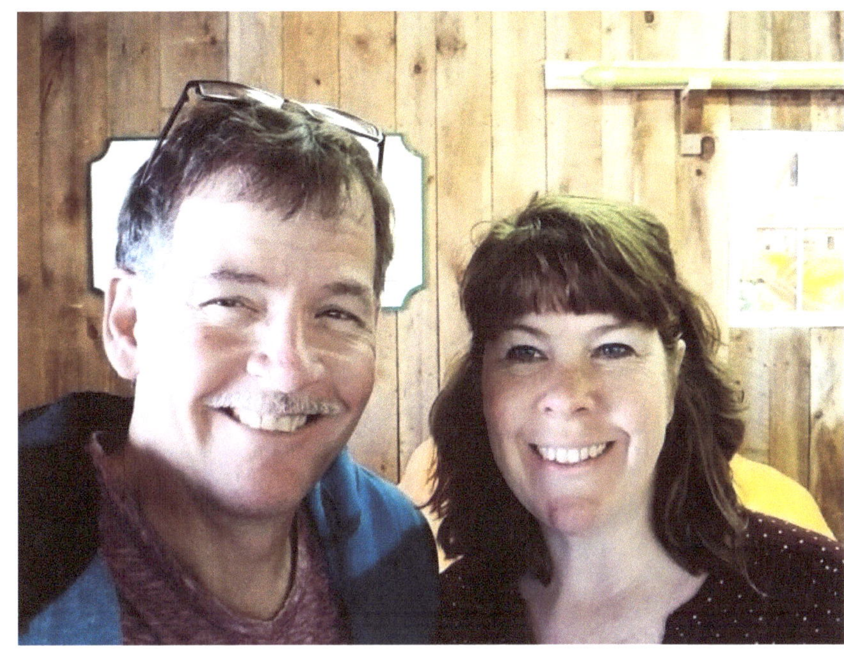

In the seven years since my own brain injury, the changes that have happened are nothing short of stunning. From the mainstream national media shining the spotlight on concussion and brain injury, to emerging technologies engineers use to diagnose brain injury, we live in exciting times.

It's hard not to look forward five, perhaps ten years ahead and wonder what other innovations will become part of the daily lives of brain injury survivors. Sometimes perspective checks are in order. Brain injury is not a new condition. If you look back to the challenges faced by survivors a few decades ago, it is hard not to be grateful, grateful that we live in a day and age where change can be seen all around us.

We hope you found something helpful to take from this month's issue.

Until next month, be well and stay strong,

~David & Sarah